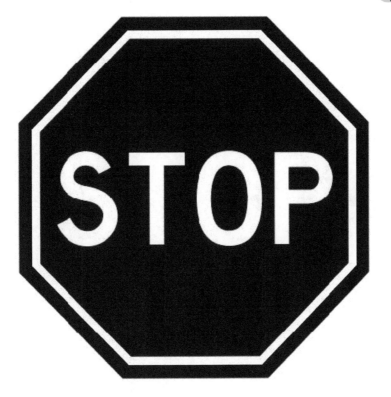

FREE Test Taking Tips DVD Offer

To help us better serve you, we have developed a Test Taking Tips DVD that we would like to give you for FREE. **This DVD covers world-class test taking tips that you can use to be even more successful when you are taking your test.**

All that we ask is that you email us your feedback about your study guide. Please let us know what you thought about it – whether that is good, bad or indifferent.

To get your **FREE Test Taking Tips DVD**, email freedvd@studyguideteam.com with "FREE DVD" in the subject line and the following information in the body of the email:

> a. The title of your study guide.
>
> b. Your product rating on a scale of 1-5, with 5 being the highest rating.
>
> c. Your feedback about the study guide. What did you think of it?
>
> d. Your full name and shipping address to send your free DVD.

If you have any questions or concerns, please don't hesitate to contact us at freedvd@studyguideteam.com.

Thanks again!

ATI TEAS 6 Study Questions 2018 & 2019

2018 & 2019

Three ATI TEAS Practice Tests Version 6

ATI TEAS Test Study Guide 2018 & 2019 Prep Team

Table of Contents

Quick Overview

As you draw closer to taking your exam, effective preparation becomes more and more important. Thankfully, you have this study guide to help you get ready. Use this guide to help keep your studying on track and refer to it often.

This study guide contains several key sections that will help you be successful on your exam. The guide contains tips for what you should do the night before and the day of the test. Also included are test-taking tips. Knowing the right information is not always enough. Many well-prepared test takers struggle with exams. These tips will help equip you to accurately read, assess, and answer test questions.

A large part of the guide is devoted to showing you what content to expect on the exam and to helping you better understand that content. Near the end of this guide is a practice test so that you can see how well you have grasped the content. Then, answer explanations are provided so that you can understand why you missed certain questions.

Don't try to cram the night before you take your exam. This is not a wise strategy for a few reasons. First, your retention of the information will be low. Your time would be better used by reviewing information you already know rather than trying to learn a lot of new information. Second, you will likely become stressed as you try to gain a large amount of knowledge in a short amount of time. Third, you will be depriving yourself of sleep. So be sure to go to bed at a reasonable time the night before. Being well-rested helps you focus and remain calm.

Be sure to eat a substantial breakfast the morning of the exam. If you are taking the exam in the afternoon, be sure to have a good lunch as well. Being hungry is distracting and can make it difficult to focus. You have hopefully spent lots of time preparing for the exam. Don't let an empty stomach get in the way of success!

When travelling to the testing center, leave earlier than needed. That way, you have a buffer in case you experience any delays. This will help you remain calm and will keep you from missing your appointment time at the testing center.

Be sure to pace yourself during the exam. Don't try to rush through the exam. There is no need to risk performing poorly on the exam just so you can leave the testing center early. Allow yourself to use all of the allotted time if needed.

Remain positive while taking the exam even if you feel like you are performing poorly. Thinking about the content you should have mastered will not help you perform better on the exam.

Once the exam is complete, take some time to relax. Even if you feel that you need to take the exam again, you will be well served by some down time before you begin studying again. It's often easier to convince yourself to study if you know that it will come with a reward!

Test-Taking Strategies

1. Predicting the Answer

When you feel confident in your preparation for a multiple-choice test, try predicting the answer before reading the answer choices. This is especially useful on questions that test objective factual knowledge or that ask you to fill in a blank. By predicting the answer before reading the available choices, you eliminate the possibility that you will be distracted or led astray by an incorrect answer choice. You will feel more confident in your selection if you read the question, predict the answer, and then find your prediction among the answer choices. After using this strategy, be sure to still read all of the answer choices carefully and completely. If you feel unprepared, you should not attempt to predict the answers. This would be a waste of time and an opportunity for your mind to wander in the wrong direction.

2. Reading the Whole Question

Too often, test takers scan a multiple-choice question, recognize a few familiar words, and immediately jump to the answer choices. Test authors are aware of this common impatience, and they will sometimes prey upon it. For instance, a test author might subtly turn the question into a negative, or he or she might redirect the focus of the question right at the end. The only way to avoid falling into these traps is to read the entirety of the question carefully before reading the answer choices.

3. Looking for Wrong Answers

Long and complicated multiple-choice questions can be intimidating. One way to simplify a difficult multiple-choice question is to eliminate all of the answer choices that are clearly wrong. In most sets of answers, there will be at least one selection that can be dismissed right away. If the test is administered on paper, the test taker could draw a line through it to indicate that it may be ignored; otherwise, the test taker will have to perform this operation mentally or on scratch paper. In either case, once the obviously incorrect answers have been eliminated, the remaining choices may be considered. Sometimes identifying the clearly wrong answers will give the test taker some information about the correct answer. For instance, if one of the remaining answer choices is a direct opposite of one of the eliminated answer choices, it may well be the correct answer. The opposite of obviously wrong is obviously right! Of course, this is not always the case. Some answers are obviously incorrect simply because they are irrelevant to the question being asked. Still, identifying and eliminating some incorrect answer choices is a good way to simplify a multiple-choice question.

4. Don't Overanalyze

Anxious test takers often overanalyze questions. When you are nervous, your brain will often run wild, causing you to make associations and discover clues that don't actually exist. If you feel that this may be a problem for you, do whatever you can to slow down during the test. Try taking a deep breath or counting to ten. As you read and consider the question, restrict yourself to the particular words used by the author. Avoid thought tangents about what the author *really* meant, or what he or she was *trying* to say. The only things that matter on a multiple-choice test are the words that are actually in the question. You must avoid reading too much into a multiple-choice question, or supposing that the writer meant something other than what he or she wrote.

5. No Need for Panic

It is wise to learn as many strategies as possible before taking a multiple-choice test, but it is likely that you will come across a few questions for which you simply don't know the answer. In this situation, avoid panicking. Because most multiple-choice tests include dozens of questions, the relative value of a single wrong answer is small. Moreover, your failure on one question has no effect on your success elsewhere on the test. As much as possible, you should compartmentalize each question on a multiple-choice test. In other words, you should not allow your feelings about one question to affect your success on the others. When you find a question that you either don't understand or don't know how to answer, just take a deep breath and do your best. Read the entire question slowly and carefully. Try rephrasing the question a couple of different ways. Then, read all of the answer choices carefully. After eliminating obviously wrong answers, make a selection and move on to the next question.

6. Confusing Answer Choices

When working on a difficult multiple-choice question, there may be a tendency to focus on the answer choices that are the easiest to understand. Many people, whether consciously or not, gravitate to the answer choices that require the least concentration, knowledge, and memory. This is a mistake. When you come across an answer choice that is confusing, you should give it extra attention. A question might be confusing because you do not know the subject matter to which it refers. If this is the case, don't eliminate the answer before you have affirmatively settled on another. When you come across an answer choice of this type, set it aside as you look at the remaining choices. If you can confidently assert that one of the other choices is correct, you can leave the confusing answer aside. Otherwise, you will need to take a moment to try to better understand the confusing answer choice. Rephrasing is one way to tease out the sense of a confusing answer choice.

7. Your First Instinct

Many people struggle with multiple-choice tests because they overthink the questions. If you have studied sufficiently for the test, you should be prepared to trust your first instinct once you have carefully and completely read the question and all of the answer choices. There is a great deal of research suggesting that the mind can come to the correct conclusion very quickly once it has obtained all of the relevant information. At times, it may seem to you as if your intuition is working faster even than your reasoning mind. This may in fact be true. The knowledge you obtain while studying may be retrieved from your subconscious before you have a chance to work out the associations that support it. Verify your instinct by working out the reasons that it should be trusted.

8. Key Words

Many test takers struggle with multiple-choice questions because they have poor reading comprehension skills. Quickly reading and understanding a multiple-choice question requires a mixture of skill and experience. To help with this, try jotting down a few key words and phrases on a piece of scrap paper. Doing this concentrates the process of reading and forces the mind to weigh the relative importance of the question's parts. In selecting words and phrases to write down, the test taker thinks about the question more deeply and carefully. This is especially true for multiple-choice questions that are preceded by a long prompt.

9. Subtle Negatives

One of the oldest tricks in the multiple-choice test writer's book is to subtly reverse the meaning of a question with a word like *not* or *except*. If you are not paying attention to each word in the question, you can easily be led astray by this trick. For instance, a common question format is, "Which of the following is...?" Obviously, if the question instead is, "Which of the following is not...?," then the answer will be quite different. Even worse, the test makers are aware of the potential for this mistake and will include one answer choice that would be correct if the question were not negated or reversed. A test taker who misses the reversal will find what he or she believes to be a correct answer and will be so confident that he or she will fail to reread the question and discover the original error. The only way to avoid this is to practice a wide variety of multiple-choice questions and to pay close attention to each and every word.

10. Reading Every Answer Choice

It may seem obvious, but you should always read every one of the answer choices! Too many test takers fall into the habit of scanning the question and assuming that they understand the question because they recognize a few key words. From there, they pick the first answer choice that answers the question they believe they have read. Test takers who read all of the answer choices might discover that one of the latter answer choices is actually *more* correct. Moreover, reading all of the answer choices can remind you of facts related to the question that can help you arrive at the correct answer. Sometimes, a misstatement or incorrect detail in one of the latter answer choices will trigger your memory of the subject and will enable you to find the right answer. Failing to read all of the answer choices is like not reading all of the items on a restaurant menu: you might miss out on the perfect choice.

11. Spot the Hedges

One of the keys to success on multiple-choice tests is paying close attention to every word. This is never more true than with words like *almost*, *most*, *some*, and *sometimes*. These words are called "hedges" because they indicate that a statement is not totally true or not true in every place and time. An absolute statement will contain no hedges, but in many subjects, like literature and history, the answers are not always straightforward or absolute. There are always exceptions to the rules in these subjects. For this reason, you should favor those multiple-choice questions that contain hedging language. The presence of qualifying words indicates that the author is taking special care with his or her words, which is certainly important when composing the right answer. After all, there are many ways to be wrong, but there is only one way to be right! For this reason, it is wise to avoid answers that are absolute when taking a multiple-choice test. An absolute answer is one that says things are either all one way or all another. They often include words like *every*, *always*, *best*, and *never*. If you are taking a multiple-choice test in a subject that doesn't lend itself to absolute answers, be on your guard if you see any of these words.

12. Long Answers

In many subject areas, the answers are not simple. As already mentioned, the right answer often requires hedges. Another common feature of the answers to a complex or subjective question are qualifying clauses, which are groups of words that subtly modify the meaning of the sentence. If the question or answer choice describes a rule to which there are exceptions or the subject matter is complicated, ambiguous, or confusing, the correct answer will require many words in order to be expressed clearly and accurately. In essence, you should not be deterred by answer choices that seem excessively long. Oftentimes, the author of the text will not be able to write the correct answer without offering some qualifications and modifications. Your job is to read the answer choices thoroughly and completely and to select the one that most accurately and precisely answers the question.

13. Restating to Understand

Sometimes, a question on a multiple-choice test is difficult not because of what it asks but because of how it is written. If this is the case, restate the question or answer choice in different words. This process serves a couple of important purposes. First, it forces you to concentrate on the core of the question. In order to rephrase the question accurately, you have to understand it well. Rephrasing the question will concentrate your mind on the key words and ideas. Second, it will present the information to your mind in a fresh way. This process may trigger your memory and render some useful scrap of information picked up while studying.

14. True Statements

Sometimes an answer choice will be true in itself, but it does not answer the question. This is one of the main reasons why it is essential to read the question carefully and completely before proceeding to the answer choices. Too often, test takers skip ahead to the answer choices and look for true statements. Having found one of these, they are content to select it without reference to the question above. Obviously, this provides an easy way for test makers to play tricks. The savvy test taker will always read the entire question before turning to the answer choices. Then, having settled on a correct answer choice, he or she will refer to the original question and ensure that the selected answer is relevant. The mistake of choosing a correct-but-irrelevant answer choice is especially common on questions related to specific pieces of objective knowledge, like historical or scientific facts. A prepared test taker will have a wealth of factual knowledge at his or her disposal, and should not be careless in its application.

15. No Patterns

One of the more dangerous ideas that circulates about multiple-choice tests is that the correct answers tend to fall into patterns. These erroneous ideas range from a belief that B and C are the most common right answers, to the idea that an unprepared test-taker should answer "A-B-A-C-A-D-A-B-A." It cannot be emphasized enough that pattern-seeking of this type is exactly the WRONG way to approach a multiple-choice test. To begin with, it is highly unlikely that the test maker will plot the correct answers according to some predetermined pattern. The questions are scrambled and delivered in a random order. Furthermore, even if the test maker was following a pattern in the assignation of correct answers, there is no reason why the test taker would know which pattern he or she was using. Any attempt to discern a pattern in the answer choices is a waste of time and a distraction from the real work of taking the test. A test taker would be much better served by extra preparation before the test than by reliance on a pattern in the answers.

FREE DVD OFFER

Don't forget that doing well on your exam includes both understanding the test content and understanding how to use what you know to do well on the test. We offer a completely FREE Test Taking Tips DVD that covers world class test taking tips that you can use to be even more successful when you are taking your test.

All that we ask is that you email us your feedback about your study guide. To get your **FREE Test Taking Tips DVD**, email freedvd@studyguideteam.com with "FREE DVD" in the subject line and the following information in the body of the email:

- The title of your study guide.
- Your product rating on a scale of 1-5, with 5 being the highest rating.
- Your feedback about the study guide. What did you think of it?
- Your full name and shipping address to send your free DVD.

Introduction to the ATI TEAS

Background of the ATI TEAS

The Test of Essential Academic Skills (TEAS) is a standardized test created and distributed by Assessment Technologies Institute (ATI) to examine the test taker's aptitude for skill sets fundamental to a career in nursing. As such, the TEAS is used by nursing schools and allied health schools in the United States and Canada as a chief criterion for admission. The TEAS is currently in its sixth iteration, known as the ATI TEAS.

The ATI TEAS is a nationwide test, with no variation in the difficulty of content among the versions given from state to state; the content of the TEAS is a standard measure for entry-level skills and abilities for nursing applicants. However, the required minimum TEAS scores, like prerequisite courses or application distinctions, can vary widely between schools and programs. Because the TEAS is used for admission to nursing and allied health programs, the majority of TEAS takers are high school diploma or GED graduates pursuing a career in nursing or are applicants to programs requiring prerequisite academic coursework. These applicants can range in background from sophomore-level collegiate to professionals looking to change careers into a healthcare field.

Test Administration

The ATI TEAS may be administered by a nursing or allied health school or a PSI testing center. The testing schedule is chosen by each individual facility, and the regularity of testing can vary from major metropolitan areas (where it may be offered multiple times per week in several locations) to sparsely populated towns (where it may be offered once per month every hundred miles). The test will also be proctored to make certain that testing protocols are enforced. Test takers can register at atitesting.com or directly through the school to which they wish to apply, as most nursing schools offer the test on-campus periodically throughout the year. The cost to take the ATI TEAS is set by the local administrator, but it usually ranges from $83 to $105.

Students may retake the ATI TEAS, but most schools have limitations such as the number of days students must wait between attempts, or the number of attempts students may make in a given period. For instance, many schools will accept the higher score of two attempts within a twelve-month period, but will not consider a third attempt until twelve months has lapsed since the first attempt. Disability accommodations are generally available and made by contacting the local test administration site.

Test Format

The ATI TEAS is comprised of 170 multiple choice questions with four possible answer choices given for each question. The questions are divided between four subject areas—Reading, Mathematics, Science, and English and Language Usage.

Subject Area	Questions	Time Limit (minutes)
Reading	53	64
Mathematics	36	54
Science	53	63
English & Language Usage	28	28
Total	**170**	**209**

Test takers are given 209 minutes to take the ATI TEAS, broken down among the four subject areas. Once a test taker begins a subject area, the timer will start. When the timer expires, the test taker may stretch, go to the bathroom, or otherwise relax before the timer begins for the next section. The ATI TEAS is offered in both a pencil-and-paper version and a computerized version, depending on the preference of the local test administrator. ATI TEAS test takers are not permitted to use cell phones, but four-function calculators are permitted now on the ATI TEAS.

Scoring

Shortly after the examination, test takers will receive several different numbered scores with their ATI TEAS results, including scores on all the various sections and subsections. This includes the national and state-level percentile rankings that a test taker has achieved. This rank is equal to the percentage of test takers from nationwide samples that scored equal to or lower than the test taker. Higher percentiles indicate more correct answers and fewer people who scored higher than the given test taker. However, although this may be of interest to the test taker, schools do not use this score to base acceptance decisions on.

Instead, schools typically look at the Composite Individual Total Score. The composite score is a good determination of the performance of the test taker and is calculated by averaging the test taker's performance from each section of the test. The national average composite score generally lies between 65% correct and 75% correct, and many schools have a minimum required score in this range, but each school and program chooses their own minimum standards; more prestigious schools require higher minimum scores and vice versa. Besides meeting minimum requirements, TEAS scores can play a part in the acceptance process as one of the factors like previous GPAs and extracurricular activities that demonstrate the competitiveness of the applicant, but this too varies from school to school.

Recent Developments

ATI TEAS is the sixth version of the TEAS, and is offered starting August 31, 2016. Before August 31, 2016, the fifth version of the TEAS (known as the TEAS V) was the current version of the TEAS. The ATI TEAS is similar in difficulty, but with slight differences in the amount of emphasis placed on various subjects, such as the reduction of the English & Language Usage section and the elimination of the Earth Science subsection. Four-function calculators are now permitted on the ATI TEAS.

ATI TEAS Practice Test #1

Reading

Questions 1–3 refer to the following paragraph.

The Brookside area is an older part of Kansas City, developed mainly in the 1920s and 30s, and is considered one of the nation's first "planned" communities with shops, restaurants, parks, and churches all within a quick walk. A stroll down any street reveals charming two-story Tudor and Colonial homes with smaller bungalows sprinkled throughout the beautiful tree-lined streets. It is common to see lemonade stands on the corners and baseball games in the numerous "pocket" parks tucked neatly behind rows of well-manicured houses. The Brookside shops on 63rd street between Wornall Road and Oak Street are a hub of commerce and entertainment where residents freely shop and dine with their pets (and children) in tow. This is also a common "hangout" spot for younger teenagers because it is easily accessible by bike for most. In short, it is an idyllic neighborhood just minutes from downtown Kansas City.

1. Which of the following states the main idea of this paragraph?
    a. The Brookside shops are a popular hangout for teenagers.
    b. There are a number of pocket parks in the Brookside neighborhood.
    c. Brookside is a great place to live.
    d. Brookside has a high crime rate.

2. In what kind of publication might you read the above paragraph?
    a. Fictional novel
    b. Community profile
    c. Newspaper article
    d. Movie review

3. According to this paragraph, which of the following is unique to this neighborhood?
    a. It is old.
    b. It is in Kansas City.
    c. It has shopping.
    d. It is one of the nation's first planned communities.

Questions 4–6 refer to the following excerpt from a government publication table of contents.

Contents

From http://purl.fdlp.gov/GPO/gpo66588

4. In which chapter would you find information for a research paper about how the nation plans to address the problem of child neglect in affected communities?
    a. Chapter 3
    b. Chapter 4
    c. Chapter 5
    d. Chapter 6

5. On which page would you find information about the needs of the American Indian child?
    a. 52
    b. 60
    c. 86
    d. 106

6. According to the table of contents, Chapter 1 is titled "Confronting the Tragedy of Child Abuse and Neglect Fatalities." Based on the chapter title and sections, which of the following is a good summary of this chapter?

a. Children's lives today are valuable and worth saving, and the children of the future are just as important.

b. The outlining of a plan to solve the problem of child neglect in disproportionately affected communities is one of the main goals here.

c. Child abuse and neglect is alive and rampant in our communities, and this chapter outlines those who are in dire need of our attention.

d. This chapter outlines resources for families who are affected by child abuse and neglect.

Questions 7–9 refer to the following excerpt taken from Walt Whitman's "Letters from a Traveling Bachelor," published in the New York Sunday Dispatch *on 14 October 1849.*

At its easternmost part, Long Island opens like the upper and under jaws of some prodigious alligator; the upper and larger one terminating in Montauk Point. The bay that lies in here, and part of which forms the splendid harbor of Greenport, where the Long Island Railroad ends, is called Peconic Bay; and a beautiful and varied water is it, fertile in fish and feathered game. I, who am by no means a skillful fisherman, go down for an hour of a morning on one of the docks, or almost anywhere along shore, and catch a mess of black-fish, which you couldn't buy in New York for a dollar—large fat fellows, with meat on their bones that it takes a pretty long fork to stick through. They have a way here of splitting these fat black-fish and poggies, and broiling them on the coals, beef-steak-fashion, which I recommend your Broadway cooks to copy.

7. Whitman's comparison of the easternmost part of Long Island to an alligator is an example of which literary device?

a. Hyperbole

b. Simile

c. Personification

d. Alliteration

8. Which of the following is the best summary of this passage?

a. Walt Whitman was impressed with the quantity and quality of fish he found in Peconic Bay.

b. Walt Whitman prefers the fish found in restaurants in New York.

c. Walt Whitman was a Broadway chef.

d. Walt Whitman is frustrated because he is not a very skilled fisherman.

9. Using the context clues in the passage, what is the meaning of the word *prodigious* in the first line?

a. Out of place

b. Great in extent, size, or degree

c. Mean-spirited

d. Extremely intelligent

10. Which of the following would be a good topic sentence if you were writing a paragraph about the effects of education on crime rates?

a. Crime statistics are difficult to verify for a number of reasons.

b. Educated people do not commit crimes.

c. Education is an important factor in lowering crime rates.

d. Education has been proven to lower crime rates by as much as 20% in some urban areas.

11. Which of the following is not an example of a good thesis statement for an essay?
   a. Animals in danger of becoming extinct come from a wide range of countries.
   b. Effective leadership requires specific qualities that anyone can develop.
   c. Industrial waste poured into Lake Michigan has killed 27 percent of marine life in the past decade.
   d. In order to fully explore the wreck of the Titanic, scientists must address several problems.

Questions 12–15 refer to the following passage, titled "Education is Essential to Civilization."

Early in my career, a master teacher shared this thought with me: "Education is the last bastion of civility." While I did not completely understand the scope of those words at the time, I have since come to realize the depth, breadth, truth, and significance of what he said. Education provides society with a vehicle for raising its children to be civil, decent, human beings with something valuable to contribute to the world. It is really what makes us human and what distinguishes us as civilized creatures.

Being "civilized" humans means being "whole" humans. Education must address the mind, body, and soul of students. It would be detrimental to society if our schools were myopic in their focus, only meeting the needs of the mind. As humans, we are multi-dimensional, multi-faceted beings who need more than head knowledge to survive. The human heart and psyche have to be fed in order for the mind to develop properly, and the body must be maintained and exercised to help fuel the working of the brain.

Education is a basic human right, and it allows us to sustain a democratic society in which participation is fundamental to its success. It should inspire students to seek better solutions to world problems and to dream of a more equitable society. Education should never discriminate on any basis, and it should create individuals who are self-sufficient, patriotic, and tolerant of other's ideas.

All children can learn, although not all children learn in the same manner. All children learn best, however, when their basic physical needs are met, and they feel safe, secure, and loved. Students are much more responsive to a teacher who values them and shows them respect as individual people. Teachers must model at all times the way they expect students to treat them and their peers. If teachers set high expectations for their students, the students will rise to that high level. Teachers must make the well-being of their students their primary focus and must not be afraid to let their students learn from their own mistakes.

In the modern age of technology, a teacher's focus is no longer the "what" of the content, but more importantly, the "why." Students are bombarded with information and have access to ANY information they need right at their fingertips. Teachers have to work harder than ever before to help students identify salient information and to think critically about the information they encounter. Students have to read between the lines, identify bias, and determine who they can trust in the milieu of ads, data, and texts presented to them.

Schools must work in consort with families in this important mission. While children spend most of their time in school, they are dramatically and indelibly shaped by the influences of their family and culture. Teachers must not only respect this fact but must strive to include parents in the education of their children and must work to keep parents informed of progress and problems. Communication between classroom and home is essential for a child's success.

Humans have always aspired to be more, do more, and to better ourselves and our communities. This is where education lies, right at the heart of humanity's desire to be all that we can be. Education helps us strive for higher goals and better treatment of ourselves and others. I shudder to think what would become of us if education ceased to be the "last bastion of civility." We must be unapologetic about expecting excellence from our students—our very existence depends upon it.

12. Which of the following best summarizes the author's main point?
    a. Education as we know it is over-valued in modern society, and we should find alternative solutions.
    b. The survival of the human race depends on the educational system, and it is worth fighting for to make it better.
    c. The government should do away with all public schools and require parents to home school their children instead.
    d. While education is important, some children simply are not capable of succeeding in a traditional classroom.

13. Based on this passage, which of the following can be inferred about the author?
    a. The author feels passionately about education.
    b. The author does not feel strongly about his point.
    c. The author is angry at the educational system.
    d. The author is unsure about the importance of education.

14. Based on this passage, which of the following conclusions could be drawn about the author?
    a. The author would not support raising taxes to help fund much needed reforms in education.
    b. The author would support raising taxes to help fund much needed reforms in education, as long as those reforms were implemented in higher socio-economic areas first.
    c. The author would support raising taxes to help fund much needed reforms in education for all children in all schools.
    d. The author would support raising taxes only in certain states to help fund much needed reforms in education.

15. According to the passage, which of the following is not mentioned as an important factor in education today?
    a. Parent involvement
    b. Communication between parents and teachers
    c. Impact of technology
    d. Cost of textbooks

For question 16, use the following graphics.

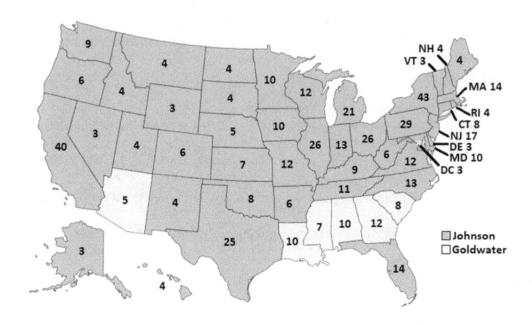

1964 Election Results			
Candidate	Party	Electoral Votes	Popular Votes
Lyndon B. Johnson	Democratic	486	42,825,463
Barry M. Goldwater	Republican	52	27,146,969

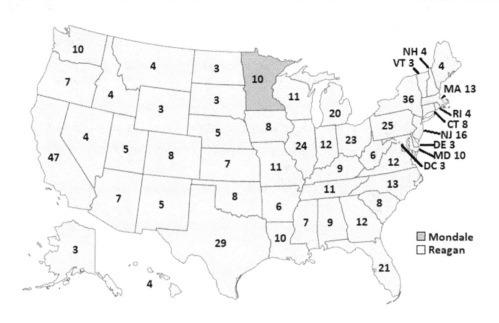

1984 Election Results			
Candidate	Party	Electoral Votes	Popular Votes
Ronald Reagan (I)	Republican	525	54,455,000
Walter F. Mondale	Democratic	13	37,577,000

16. Based on the two maps, which of the following statements is true?
    a. Over twenty years, the country's voter turnout for a presidential election stayed the exact same.
    b. Over twenty years, there was a noticeable decrease in voter turnout during a presidential election.
    c. Over twenty years, the electoral vote swung from almost completely Democrat to almost completely Republican.
    d. There was very little change in the number of electoral votes won for each party from 1964 to 1984.

For question 17, use the following graphic.

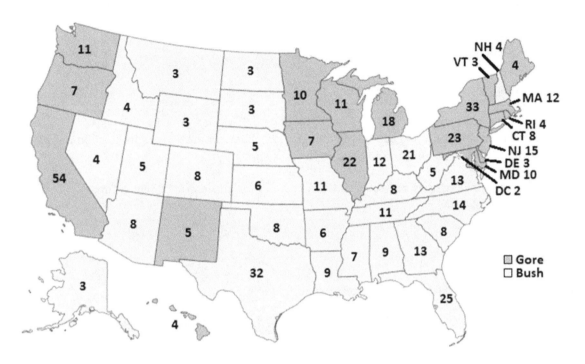

2000 Election Results			
Candidate	Party	Electoral Votes	Popular Votes
George W. Bush	Republican	271	50,456,062
Albert Gore, Jr.	Democratic	266	50,996,582

17. Based on the map, which of the following statements is NOT true?
    a. In 2000, the Democratic candidate won the popular vote, which means he won more the electoral votes of more states.
    b. In 2000, the Republican candidate won the presidential election because he won the electoral vote even though he did not win the popular vote.
    c. In 2000, the Democratic candidate won the popular vote but not the electoral vote, which reveals a discrepancy in the electoral system.
    d. In 2000, the Republican candidate won more states but did not win the popular vote.

18. If you were asked to write a comprehensive research paper about life during the Great Depression in United States, which of the following would be a reliable primary source?

    a. Wikipedia article titled "Life in Depression America."

    b. Diary entry from Elsie May Long published in the article "The Great Depression: Two Kansas Diaries" by C. Robert Haywood in *Great Plains Quarterly*.

    c. Article titled "The Great Depression Begins: the Stock Market Crash of 1929," found at http://www.history.com/topics/great-depression

    d. Book by Glen H. Elder, Jr. titled *Children of the Great Depressions: Social Change in Life Experience*, published in 1999 by the American Psychological Association.

19. "Excuse me, Sir," the host of the party declared, "this matter is not *any* of your business." The use of italics in this sentence indicates which of the following?

    a. Dialogue

    b. Thoughts

    c. Emphasis

    d. Volume

20. Snails, clams, mussels, and squid are mollusks, i.e., invertebrates with soft, unsegmented bodies that live in aquatic or damp habitats and have calcareous shells.

Which of the following does the abbreviation i.e. stand for in the preceding sentence?

    a. For example

    b. In error

    c. In addition

    d. That is

Questions 21–23 are based upon the following passage:

This excerpt is adaptation from Charles Dickens' speech in Birmingham in England on December 30, 1853 on behalf of the Birmingham and Midland Institute.

> My Good Friends,—When I first imparted to the committee of the projected Institute my particular wish that on one of the evenings of my readings here the main body of my audience should be composed of working men and their families, I was animated by two desires; first, by the wish to have the great pleasure of meeting you face to face at this Christmas time, and accompany you myself through one of my little Christmas books; and second, by the wish to have an opportunity of stating publicly in your presence, and in the presence of the committee, my earnest hope that the Institute will, from the beginning, recognise one great principle—strong in reason and justice—which I believe to be essential to the very life of such an Institution. It is, that the working man shall, from the first unto the last, have a share in the management of an Institution which is designed for his benefit, and which calls itself by his name.

> I have no fear here of being misunderstood—of being supposed to mean too much in this. If there ever was a time when any one class could of itself do much for its own good, and for the welfare of society—which I greatly doubt—that time is unquestionably past. It is in the fusion of different classes, without confusion; in the bringing together of employers and employed; in the creating of a better common understanding among those whose interests are identical, who depend upon each

other, who are vitally essential to each other, and who never can be in unnatural antagonism without deplorable results, that one of the chief principles of a Mechanics' Institution should consist. In this world a great deal of the bitterness among us arises from an imperfect understanding of one another. Erect in Birmingham a great Educational Institution, properly educational; educational of the feelings as well as of the reason; to which all orders of Birmingham men contribute; in which all orders of Birmingham men meet; wherein all orders of Birmingham men are faithfully represented—and you will erect a Temple of Concord here which will be a model edifice to the whole of England.

Contemplating as I do the existence of the Artisans' Committee, which not long ago considered the establishment of the Institute so sensibly, and supported it so heartily, I earnestly entreat the gentlemen—earnest I know in the good work, and who are now among us,—by all means to avoid the great shortcoming of similar institutions; and in asking the working man for his confidence, to set him the great example and give him theirs in return. You will judge for yourselves if I promise too much for the working man, when I say that he will stand by such an enterprise with the utmost of his patience, his perseverance, sense, and support; that I am sure he will need no charitable aid or condescending patronage; but will readily and cheerfully pay for the advantages which it confers; that he will prepare himself in individual cases where he feels that the adverse circumstances around him have rendered it necessary; in a word, that he will feel his responsibility like an honest man, and will most honestly and manfully discharge it. I now proceed to the pleasant task to which I assure you I have looked forward for a long time.

21. Based upon the contextual evidence provided in the passage above, what is the meaning of the term *enterprise* in the third paragraph?
    a. Company
    b. Courage
    c. Game
    d. Cause

22. The speaker addresses his audience as *My Good Friends*—what kind of credibility does this salutation give to the speaker?
    a. The speaker is an employer addressing his employees, so the salutation is a way for the boss to bridge the gap between himself and his employees.
    b. The speaker's salutation is one from an entertainer to his audience and uses the friendly language to connect to his audience before a serious speech.
    c. The salutation gives the serious speech that follows a somber tone, as it is used ironically.
    d. The speech is one from a politician to the public, so the salutation is used to grab the audience's attention.

23. According to the aforementioned passage, what is the speaker's second desire for his time in front of the audience?
    a. To read a Christmas story
    b. For the working man to have a say in his institution which is designed for his benefit.
    c. To have an opportunity to stand in their presence
    d. For the life of the institution to be essential to the audience as a whole

Use the following image to answer questions 9 and 10.

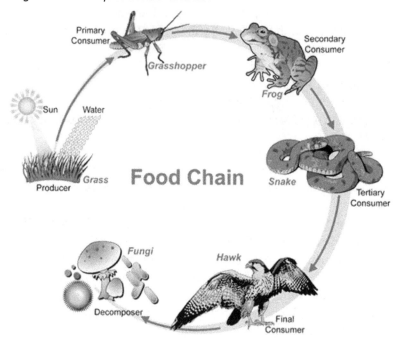

24. Which is the decomposer in the food chain above?
    a. Sun
    b. Grass
    c. Frog
    d. Fungi

25. Which is the herbivore in the food chain above?
    a. Grass
    b. Grasshopper
    c. Frog
    d. Fungi

26. Consider the following headings that might be found under the entry for "Basketball" in an electronic encyclopedia.

  ▪ Introduction
  ▪ Basic Rules
  ▪ Professional Basketball
  ▪ College Basketball
  ▪ Similarities to Lacrosse
  ▪ Olympic and International Basketball
  ▪ Women's Basketball
  ▪ Bibliography

Which one does not belong?
    a. Women's Basketball
    b. Similarities to Lacrosse
    c. Basic Rules
    d. Bibliography

27. The guidewords at the top of a dictionary page are *receipt* and *reveal*. Which of the following words is NOT an entry on this page?

    a. Receive

    b. Retail

    c. Revere

    d. Reluctant

Use the nutrition label below for questions 28–30.

Nutrition Facts

Serving Size 2/3 cup (55g)
Servings Per Container About 8

Amount Per Serving

Calories 230   Calories from Fat 72

	% Daily Value*
Total Fat 8g	**12%**
Saturated Fat 1g	**5%**
Trans Fat 0g	
Cholesterol 0mg	**0%**
Sodium 160mg	**7%**
Total Carbohydrate 37g	**12%**
Dietary Fiber 4g	**16%**
Sugars 1g	
Protein 3g	
Vitamin A	10%
Vitamin C	8%
Calcium	20%
Iron	45%

* Percent Daily Values are based on a 2,000 calorie diet. Your daily value may be higher or lower depending on your calorie needs.

	Calories:	2,000	2,500
Total Fat	Less than	65g	80g
Sat Fat	Less than	20g	25g
Cholesterol	Less than	300mg	300mg
Sodium	Less than	2,400mg	2,400mg
Total Carbohydrate		300g	375g
Dietary Fiber		25g	30g

28. Based on the information provided on the nutrition label, approximately what percent of the total calories come from fat?

    a. 12%

    b. 33%

    c. 5%

    d. 0%

29. If Alex ate two cups of this product, approximately how many calories did he consume?

    a. Almost 700 calories

    b. A little more than 200 calories

    c. Around 450 calories

    d. A little more than 70

30. Based on the information from the nutrition label above, which of the following statements is true?
    a. Someone eating this food item would not need to worry for the rest of the day about getting more of vitamins A and C.
    b. This food item is not a good source of iron.
    c. For someone consuming 2,000 calories a day, this food item contains too much dietary fiber.
    d. Someone on a low sodium diet would not need to worry about this food item being high in sodium.

31. In her famous poem "Because I Could Not Stop for Death," Emily Dickinson writes, "Because I could not stop for Death / He kindly stopped for me." Her mention of death is an example of which of the following?
    a. Hyperbole
    b. Personification
    c. Allusion
    d. Alliteration

32. In the poem quoted above, what does the slash mark between the words "Death" and "He" represent?
    a. The break between two stanzas
    b. The end of one sentence and the start of another
    c. The break between two lines of poetry
    d. The shift from one speaker to another

Use the following three quotations from Thomas Jefferson to answer questions 33 and 34.

"The tree of liberty must be refreshed from time to time with the blood of patriots and tyrants."

"In matters of style, swim with the current; in matters of principle, stand like a rock."

"I hold it, that a little rebellion, now and then, is a good thing, and as necessary in the political world as storms in the physical."

33. What is Jefferson's opinion on conflict?
    a. It is unavoidable and necessary.
    b. It must be avoided at all costs.
    c. Staying true to your principles is never worth the price you might pay.
    d. It will lead to ultimate destruction.

34. The "tree of liberty" is an example of which of the following?
    a. Personification
    b. Allusion
    c. Analogy
    d. Idiom

35. If you were looking for the most reliable and up-to-date information regarding the safety of travel overseas, which of the following websites would be the most accurate?
    a. http://www.nomadicmatt.com/travel-blog/
    b. https://en.wikipedia.org/wiki/Tourism
    c. http://gizmodo.com/how-to-travel-internationally-for-the-very-first-time
    d. http://www.state.gov/travel/

Use the following excerpt for questions 36 and 37.

Evidently, our country has overlooked both the importance of learning history and the appreciation of it. But why is this a huge problem? Other than historians, who really cares how the War of 1812 began, or who Alexander the Great's tutor was? Well, not many, as it turns out. So, *is* history really that important? Yes! History is **critical** to help us understand the underlying forces that shape decisive events, to prevent us from making the same mistakes twice, and to give us context for current events.

36. The above is an example of which type of writing?
    a. Expository
    b. Persuasive
    c. Narrative
    d. Poetry

37. In the above passage, what does the use of boldface type for the word "critical" indicate?
    a. Dialogue
    b. Volume
    c. Emphasis
    d. Misspelling

38. The guidewords at the top of a dictionary page are *able-bodied* and *about-face*. Which of the following words appear as an entry on this page?
    a. Abolition
    b. Abundant
    c. Able
    d. Ability

39. Synonyms of the word *spurious* are *feigned* and *fraudulent*. Which of the following is an antonym for *spurious*?
    a. Phony
    b. Impersonated
    c. Misleading
    d. Genuine

40. Which of the following sentences contains an opinion statement?
    a. In 1819, the Supreme Court ruled that Congress could create a national bank.
    b. Marshall also ruled that the states did not have the right to tax the bank or any other agency created by the federal government.
    c. John Marshall was one of the most intelligent chief justices in the United States.
    d. The chief justice is the head of the judicial branch of the government.

41. Which of the following sentences is a factual statement?
    a. Many nutritionists believe a low carbohydrate, high protein diet is the healthiest diet.
    b. Legislation should be passed mandating that cell phones be banned in all public-school classrooms.
    c. Spanish is an easier language to learn than Japanese.
    d. College students would benefit greatly from participating in intramural sports on their campuses.

42. Follow the numbered instructions to transform the starting word into a different word.

1. Start with the word *CARLOAD*.
2. Move the first letter to the end of the word.
3. Switch the first and second letters.
4. Switch the third and sixth letters.
5. Change the fourth letter to an *i*.
6. Move the last letter before the second *a*.

What is the new word?
   a. Carpool
   b. Radical
   c. Ordeal
   d. Railroad

Questions 43 and 44 refer to the following quote from Martin Luther King Jr.'s Nobel Peace Prize acceptance speech in Oslo on December 10, 1964.

> "I refuse to accept the view that mankind is so tragically bound to the starless midnight of racism and war that the bright daybreak of peace and brotherhood can never become a reality . . . I believe that unarmed truth and unconditional love will have the final word."

43. Which of the following statements is NOT accurate based on this quote?
   a. Martin Luther King Jr. felt that the fight against racism was ultimately hopeless due to mankind's primitive instincts.
   b. Martin Luther King Jr. was eternally optimistic about mankind's ability to overcome racism.
   c. Martin Luther King Jr. believed that the war against racism could be won with truth and love.
   d. Martin Luther King Jr. believed in that the goodness of mankind would prevail.

44. By referring to the "starless midnight of racism," Martin Luther King means:
   a. Racism involves prejudices against people with dark skin.
   b. Racism is evil and blinds people to the truth.
   c. It is easier to be racist on a starless night.
   d. The problem of racism is not as bad during the day.

Questions 45–48 refer to the following passage.

> Although many Missourians know that Harry S. Truman and Walt Disney hailed from their great state, probably far fewer know that it was also home to the remarkable George Washington Carver. At the end of the Civil War, Moses Carver, the slave owner who owned George's parents, decided to keep George and his brother and raise them on his farm. As a child, George was driven to learn and he loved painting. He even went on to study art while in college but was encouraged to pursue botany instead. He spent much of his life helping others by showing them better ways to farm; his ideas improved agricultural productivity in many countries. One of his most notable contributions to the newly emerging class of Negro farmers was to teach them the negative effects of agricultural monoculture, i.e. growing the same crops in the same fields year after year, depleting the soil of much needed nutrients and resulting in a lesser yielding crop. Carver was an innovator, always thinking of new and better ways to do things, and is most famous for his over three hundred uses for the peanut. Toward the end of his career, Carver returned to his first love of art. Through his artwork, he hoped to inspire people to see the

beauty around them and to do great things themselves. When Carver died, he left his money to help fund ongoing agricultural research. Today, people still visit and study at the George Washington Carver Foundation at Tuskegee Institute.

45. Which of the following describes the kind of writing used in the above passage?
    a. Narrative
    b. Persuasive
    c. Technical
    d. Expository

46. According to the passage, what was George Washington Carver's first love?
    a. Plants
    b. Art
    c. Animals
    d. Soil

47. According to the passage, what is the best definition for agricultural monoculture?
    a. The practice of producing or growing a single crop or plant species over a wide area and for a large number of consecutive years
    b. The practice of growing a diversity of crops and rotating them from year to year
    c. The practice of growing crops organically to avoid the use of pesticides
    d. The practice of charging an inflated price for cheap crops to obtain a greater profit margin

48. Which of the following is the best summary of this passage?
    a. George Washington Carver was born at a time when scientific discovery was at a virtual standstill.
    b. Because he was African American, there were not many opportunities for George Washington Carver.
    c. George Washington Carver was an intelligent man whose research and discoveries had an impact worldwide.
    d. George Washington Carver was far more successful as an artist than he was as a scientist.

Questions 49–53 are based upon the following passage:

This excerpt is adaptation from *The Life-Story of Insects,* by Geo H. Carpenter.

> Insects as a whole are preeminently creatures of the land and the air. This is shown not only by the possession of wings by a vast majority of the class, but by the mode of breathing to which reference has already been made, a system of branching air-tubes carrying atmospheric air with its combustion-supporting oxygen to all the insect's tissues. The air gains access to these tubes through a number of paired air-holes or spiracles, arranged segmentally in series.
>
> It is of great interest to find that, nevertheless, a number of insects spend much of their time under water. This is true of not a few in the perfect winged state, as for example aquatic beetles and water-bugs ('boatmen' and 'scorpions') which have some way of protecting their spiracles when submerged, and, possessing usually the power of flight, can pass on occasion from pond or stream to upper air. But it is advisable in connection with our present subject to dwell especially on some insects that remain continually under water till they are ready to undergo their final moult and attain the winged state, which they pass entirely in the air. The preparatory instars of such insects are aquatic;

the adult instar is aerial. All may-flies, dragon-flies, and caddis-flies, many beetles and two-winged flies, and a few moths thus divide their life-story between the water and the air. For the present we confine attention to the Stone-flies, the May-flies, and the Dragon-flies, three well-known orders of insects respectively called by systematists the Plecoptera, the Ephemeroptera and the Odonata.

In the case of many insects that have aquatic larvae, the latter are provided with some arrangement for enabling them to reach atmospheric air through the surface-film of the water. But the larva of a stone-fly, a dragon-fly, or a may-fly is adapted more completely than these for aquatic life; it can, by means of gills of some kind, breathe the air dissolved in water.

49. Which statement best details the central idea in this passage?
    a. It introduces certain insects that transition from water to air.
    b. It delves into entomology, especially where gills are concerned.
    c. It defines what constitutes as insects' breathing.
    d. It invites readers to have a hand in the preservation of insects.

50. Which definition most closely relates to the usage of the word *moult* in the passage?
    a. An adventure of sorts, especially underwater
    b. Mating act between two insects
    c. The act of shedding part or all of the outer shell
    d. Death of an organism that ends in a revival of life

51. What is the purpose of the first paragraph in relation to the second paragraph?
    a. The first paragraph serves as a cause and the second paragraph serves as an effect.
    b. The first paragraph serves as a contrast to the second.
    c. The first paragraph is a description for the argument in the second paragraph.
    d. The first and second paragraphs are merely presented in a sequence.

52. What does the following sentence most nearly mean?
    The preparatory instars of such insects are aquatic; the adult instar is aerial.

    a. The volume of water is necessary to prep the insect for transition rather than the volume of the air.
    b. The abdomen of the insect is designed like a star in the water as well as the air.
    c. The stage of preparation in between molting is acted out in the water, while the last stage is in the air.
    d. These insects breathe first in the water through gills yet continue to use the same organs to breathe in the air.

53. Which of the statements reflect information that one could reasonably infer based on the author's tone?
    a. The author's tone is persuasive and attempts to call the audience to action.
    b. The author's tone is passionate due to excitement over the subject and personal narrative.
    c. The author's tone is informative and exhibits interest in the subject of the study.
    d. The author's tone is somber, depicting some anger at the state of insect larvae.

Math

1. Which of the following is largest?
    a. 0.45
    b. 0.096
    c. 0.3
    d. 0.313

2. Which of the following is NOT a way to write 40 percent of N?
    a. $(0.4)N$

    b. $\frac{2}{5}N$

    c. $40N$

    d. $\frac{4N}{10}$

3. Which is closest to 17.8×9.9?
    a. 140
    b. 180
    c. 200
    d. 350

4. A student gets an 85% on a test with 20 questions. How many answers did the student solve correctly?
    a. 15
    b. 16
    c. 17
    d. 18

5. Four people split a bill. The first person pays for $\frac{1}{5}$, the second person pays for $\frac{1}{4}$, and the third person pays for $\frac{1}{3}$. What fraction of the bill does the fourth person pay?
    a. $\frac{13}{60}$

    b. $\frac{47}{60}$

    c. $\frac{1}{4}$

    d. $\frac{4}{15}$

6. 6 is 30% of what number?
    a. 18
    b. 20
    c. 24
    d. 26

7. $3\frac{2}{3} - 1\frac{4}{5} =$

    a. $1\frac{13}{15}$

    b. $\frac{14}{15}$

    c. $2\frac{2}{3}$

    d. $\frac{4}{5}$

8. What is $\frac{420}{98}$ rounded to the nearest integer?

    a. 4
    b. 3
    c. 5
    d. 6

9. $4\frac{1}{3} + 3\frac{3}{4} =$

    a. $6\frac{5}{12}$

    b. $8\frac{1}{12}$

    c. $8\frac{2}{3}$

    d. $7\frac{7}{12}$

10. Five of six numbers have a sum of 25. The average of all six numbers is 6. What is the sixth number?

    a. 8
    b. 10
    c. 11
    d. 12

11. $52.3 \times 10^{-3} =$

    a. 0.00523
    b. 0.0523
    c. 0.523
    d. 523

12. If $\frac{5}{2} \div \frac{1}{3} = n$, then n is between:

    a. 5 and 7
    b. 7 and 9
    c. 9 and 11
    d. 3 and 5

13. A closet is filled with red, blue, and green shirts. If $\frac{1}{3}$ of the shirts are green and $\frac{2}{5}$ are red, what fraction of the shirts are blue?

    a. $\frac{4}{15}$

    b. $\frac{1}{5}$

    c. $\frac{7}{15}$

    d. $\frac{1}{2}$

14. Shawna buys $2\frac{1}{2}$ gallons of paint. If she uses $\frac{1}{3}$ of it on the first day, how much does she have left?

    a. $1\frac{5}{6}$ gallons

    b. $1\frac{1}{2}$ gallons

    c. $1\frac{2}{3}$ gallons

    d. 2 gallons

15. What is the value of $x^2 - 2xy + 2y^2$ when $x = 2, y = 3$?
    a. 8
    b. 10
    c. 12
    d. 14

16. $(2x - 4y)^2 =$
    a. $4x^2 - 16xy + 16y^2$
    b. $4x^2 - 8xy + 16y^2$
    c. $4x^2 - 16xy - 16y^2$
    d. $2x^2 - 8xy + 8y^2$

17. On Monday, Robert mopped the floor in 4 hours. On Tuesday, he did it in 3 hours. If on Monday, his average rate of mopping was p sq. ft. per hour, what was his average rate on Tuesday?

    a. $\frac{4}{3}p$ sq. ft. per hour

    b. $\frac{3}{4}p$ sq. ft. per hour

    c. $\frac{5}{4}p$ sq. ft. per hour

    d. $p + 1$ sq. ft. per hour

18. The variable y is directly proportional to x. If $y = 3$ when $x = 5$, then what is y when $x = 20$?
    a. 10
    b. 12
    c. 14
    d. 16

19. There are $4x + 1$ treats in each party favor bag. If a total of $60x + 15$ treats are distributed, how many bags are given out?

    a. 15

    b. 16

    c. 20

    d. 22

20. Apples cost $2 each, while oranges cost $3 each. Maria purchased 10 fruits in total and spent $22. How many apples did she buy?

    a. 5

    b. 6

    c. 7

    d. 8

21. A rectangle has a length that is 5 feet longer than three times its width. If the perimeter is 90 feet, what is the length in feet?

    a. 10

    b. 20

    c. 25

    d. 35

22. Five students take a test. The scores of the first four students are 80, 85, 75, and 60. If the median score is 80, which of the following could NOT be the score of the fifth student?

    a. 60

    b. 80

    c. 85

    d. 100

23. In an office, there are 50 workers. A total of 60% of the workers are women, and the chances of a woman wearing a skirt is 50%. If no men wear skirts, how many workers are wearing skirts?

    a. 12

    b. 15

    c. 16

    d. 20

24. Ten students take a test. Five students get a 50. Four students get a 70. If the average score is 55, what was the last student's score?

    a. 20

    b. 40

    c. 50

    d. 60

25. A company invests $50,000 in a building where they can produce saws. If the cost of producing one saw is $40, then which function expresses the amount of money the company pays? The variable y is the money paid and x is the number of saws produced.

    a. $y = 50,000x + 40$

    b. $y + 40 = x - 50,000$

    c. $y = 40x - 50,000$

    d. $y = 40x + 50,000$

26. A six-sided die is rolled. What is the probability that the roll is 1 or 2?

    a. $\frac{1}{6}$

    b. $\frac{1}{4}$

    c. $\frac{1}{3}$

    d. $\frac{1}{2}$

27. An equilateral triangle has a perimeter of 18 feet. If a square whose sides have the same length as one side of the triangle is built, what will be the area of the square?

    a. 6 square feet
    b. 36 square feet
    c. 256 square feet
    d. 1000 square feet

28. Mom's car drove 72 miles in 90 minutes. How fast did she drive in feet per second?

    a. 0.8 feet per second
    b. 48.9 feet per second
    c. 0.009 feet per second
    d. 70. 4 feet per second

29. How do you solve $V = lwh$ for h?

    a. $lwV = h$

    b. $h = \frac{V}{lw}$

    c. $h = \frac{Vl}{w}$

    d. $h = \frac{Vw}{l}$

30. If Sarah reads at an average rate of 21 pages in four nights, how long will it take her to read 140 pages?

    a. 6 nights
    b. 26 nights
    c. 8 nights
    d. 27 nights

31. The phone bill is calculated each month using the equation $c = 50g + 75$. The cost of the phone bill per month is represented by c, and g represents the gigabytes of data used that month. What is the value and interpretation of the slope of this equation?

    a. 75 dollars per day
    b. 75 gigabytes per day
    c. 50 dollars per day
    d. 50 dollars per gigabyte

32. Twenty is 40% of what number?
    a. 50
    b. 8
    c. 200
    d. 5000

33. What is the volume of a cube with the side equal to 3 inches?
    a. 6 in³
    b. 27 in³
    c. 9 in³
    d. 3 in³

34. What is the volume of a cube with the side equal to 5 centimeters?
    a. 10 cm³
    b. 15 cm³
    c. 50 cm³
    d. 125 cm³

35. What is the volume of a rectangular prism with a height of 2 inches, a width of 4 inches, and a depth of 6 inches?
    a. 12 in³
    b. 24 in³
    c. 48 in³
    d. 96 in³

36. What is the volume of a rectangular prism with the height of 3 centimeters, a width of 5 centimeters, and a depth of 11 centimeters?
    a. 19 cm³
    b. 165 cm³
    c. 225 cm³
    d. 150 cm³

Science

1. What is the total mechanical energy of a system?
    a. The total potential energy
    b. The total kinetic energy
    c. Kinetic energy plus potential energy
    d. Kinetic energy minus potential energy

2. What does the Lewis Dot structure of an element represent?
    a. The outer electron valence shell population
    b. The inner electron valence shell population
    c. The positioning of the element's protons
    d. The positioning of the element's neutrons

3. What is the name of the scale used in sound level meters to measure the intensity of sound waves?
    a. Doppler
    b. Electron
    c. Watt
    d. Decibel

4. Which statement is true regarding electrostatic charges?
    a. Like charges attract.
    b. Like charges repel.
    c. Like charges are neutral.
    d. Like charges neither attract nor repel.

5. In which organelle do eukaryotes carry out aerobic respiration?
    a. Golgi apparatus
    b. Nucleus
    c. Mitochondrion
    d. Cytosol

6. What kind of energy do plants use in photosynthesis to create chemical energy?
    a. Light
    b. Electric
    c. Nuclear
    d. Cellular

7. What type of biological molecule is a monosaccharide?
    a. Protein
    b. Carbohydrate
    c. Nucleic acid
    d. Lipid

8. Which level of protein structure is defined by the folds and coils of the protein's polypeptide backbone?
    a. Primary
    b. Secondary
    c. Tertiary
    d. Quaternary

9. A scientist is trying to determine how much poison will kill a rat the fastest. Which of the following statements is an example of an appropriate hypothesis?
    a. Rats that are given lots of poison seem to die quickly.
    b. Does the amount of poison affect how quickly the rat dies?
    c. The more poison a rat is given, the quicker it will die.
    d. Poison is fatal to rats.

10. In testing how quickly a rat dies by the amount of poison it eats, which of the following is the independent variable and which is the dependent variable?

    a. How quickly the rat dies is the independent variable; the amount of poison is the dependent variable.

    b. The amount of poison is the independent variable; how quickly the rat dies is the dependent variable.

    c. Whether the rat eats the poison is the independent variable; how quickly the rat dies is the dependent variable.

    d. The cage the rat is kept in is the independent variable; the amount of poison is the dependent variable.

11. Which of the following is a representation of a natural pattern or occurrence that's difficult or impossible to experience directly?

    a. A theory

    b. A model

    c. A law

    d. An observation

12. Which of the following is a standard or series of standards to which the results from an experiment are compared?

    a. A control

    b. A variable

    c. A constant

    d. Collected data

13. "This flower is dead; someone must have forgotten to water it." This statement is an example of which of the following?

    a. A classification

    b. An observation

    c. An inference

    d. A collection

14. How many centimeters is 0.78 kilometers?

    a. 7.8 cm

    b. 0.078 cm

    c. 78,000 cm

    d. 780 cm

15. 4.67 miles is equivalent to how many kilometers to three significant digits?

    a. 7.514 km

    b. 7.51 km

    c. 2.90 km

    d. 2.902 km

16. When considering anatomical direction, what is the position of the clavicle to the humerus?

    a. Lateral

    b. Medial

    c. Distal

    d. Inferior

17. What is the body plane that runs vertically through the body at right angles to the midline?
    a. Coronal
    b. Transverse
    c. Sagittal
    d. Superior

18. Which statement is true?
    a. Ligaments attach skeletal muscles to bone.
    b. Tendons connect bones at joints.
    c. Cartilage adds mechanical support to joints.
    d. Most veins deliver oxygenated blood to cells.

19. Which layer of skin contains sensory receptors and blood vessels?
    a. Epidermis
    b. Dermis
    c. Hypodermis
    d. Subcutaneous

20. What locations in the digestive system are sites of chemical digestion?
    I.   Mouth
    II.   Stomach
    III. Small Intestine
    a. II only
    b. III only
    c. II and III only
    d. I, II, and III only

21. The radius and ulna are to the humerus what the tibia and fibula are to the _____.
    a. Mandible
    b. Femur
    c. Scapula
    d. Carpal

22. What are concentric circles of bone tissue are called?
    a. Lacunae
    b. Lamellae
    c. Trabeculae
    d. Diaphysis

23. When de-oxygenated blood first enters the heart, which of the following choices is in the correct order for its journey to the aorta?
    I. Tricuspid valve → Lungs → Mitral valve
    II. Mitral valve → Lungs → Tricuspid valve
    III. Right ventricle → Lungs → Left atrium
    IV. Left ventricle → Lungs → Right atrium
    a. I and III only
    b. I and IV only
    c. II and III only
    d. II and IV only

24. Which characteristics are true for skeletal muscle?
    I. Contain sarcomeres
    II. Have multiple nuclei
    III. Are branched
    a. I only
    b. I and II only
    c. I, II, and III only
    d. II and III only

25. Which is the simplest nerve pathway that bypasses the brain?
    a. Autonomic
    b. Reflex arc
    c. Somatic
    d. Sympathetic

26. What is the order of filtration in the nephron?
    a. Collecting Duct → Proximal tubule → Loop of Henle
    b. Proximal tubule → Loop of Henle → Collecting duct
    c. Loop of Henle → Collecting duct → Proximal tubule
    d. Loop of Henle → Proximal tubule → Collecting duct

27. Which function below corresponds to the parasympathetic nervous system?
    a. Stimulates the fight-or-flight response
    b. Increases heart rate
    c. Stimulates digestion
    d. Increases bronchiole dilation

28. Which are neurons that transmit signals from the CNS to effector tissues and organs?
    a. Motor
    b. Sensory
    c. Interneuron
    d. Reflex

29. Which statement is NOT true regarding brain structure?
    a. The corpus collosum connects the hemispheres.
    b. Broca and Wernicke's areas are associated with speech and language.
    c. The cerebellum is important for long-term memory storage.
    d. The brainstem is responsible for involuntary movement.

30. Which is NOT a function of the pancreas?
    a. Secretes the hormone insulin in response to growth hormone stimulation
    b. Secretes bicarbonate into the small intestine to raise the pH from stomach secretions
    c. Secretes enzymes used by the small intestine to digest fats, sugars, and proteins
    d. Secretes hormones from its endocrine portion in order to regulate blood sugar levels

31. Which organ is not a component of the lymphatic system?
    a. Thymus
    b. Spleen
    c. Tonsil
    d. Gall bladder

32. Which action is unrelated to blood pH?
    a. Exhalation of carbon dioxide
    b. Kidney reabsorption of bicarbonate
    c. ADH secretion
    d. Nephron secretion of ammonia

33. Which gland regulates calcium levels?
    a. Thyroid
    b. Pineal
    c. Adrenal
    d. Parathyroid

34. What are the functions of the hypothalamus?
    I. Regulate body temperature
    II. Send stimulatory and inhibitory instructions to the pituitary gland
    III. Receives sensory information from the brain
    a. I and II
    b. I and III
    c. II and III
    d. I, II, and III

35. Which muscle system is unlike the others?
    a. Bicep: Tricep
    b. Quadricep: Hamstring
    c. Gluteus maximus: Gluteus minimus
    d. Trapezius/Rhomboids: Pectoralis Major

36. Which blood component is chiefly responsible for clotting?
    a. Platelets
    b. Red blood cells
    c. Antigens
    d. Plasma cells

37. Which is the first event to happen in a primary immune response?
    a. Macrophages phagocytose pathogens and present their antigens.
    b. Neutrophils aggregate and act as cytotoxic, nonspecific killers of pathogens.
    c. B lymphocytes make pathogen-specific antibodies.
    d. Helper T cells secrete interleukins to activate pathogen-fighting cells.

38. Where does sperm maturation take place in the male reproductive system?
    a. Seminal vesicles
    b. Prostate gland
    c. Epididymis
    d. Vas Deferens

39. Which hormone in the female reproductive system is responsible for progesterone production?
    a. FSH
    b. LH
    c. hCG
    d. Estrogen

40. Which epithelial tissue comprises the cell layer found in a capillary bed?
    a. Squamous
    b. Cuboidal
    c. Columnar
    d. Stratified

41. How do muscle fibers shorten during contraction?
    a. The actin filaments attach to the myosin forming cross-bridges and pull the fibers closer together
    b. Calcium enters the sarcoplasmic reticulum, initiating an action potential
    c. Myosin cross-bridges attach, rotate, and detach from actin filaments causing the ends of the sarcomere to be pulled closer together
    d. The t-tubule system allows the fibers to physically shorten during contraction

42. Which of the following is not considered to be a primary function of the proprioceptive system?
    a. Provide awareness of position and kinesthesia within the surroundings
    b. Produce coordinated reflexes to maintain muscle tone and balance
    c. Provide peripheral feedback information to the central nervous system to help modify movements and motor response
    d. Provide cushioning to joints during impact

43. Which of the following correctly explain the order of how muscle spindles sense the rate and magnitude of increasing muscle tension as the muscle lengthens?
    a. The muscle spindle is stretched, sensory neurons in the spindle are activated, an impulse is sent to the spinal cord, motor neurons that innervate extrafusal fibers are signaled to relax
    b. The muscle spindle is stretched, motor neurons in the spindle are activated, an impulse is sent to the spinal cord, sensory neurons that innervate extrafusal fibers are signaled to relax
    c. Sensory neurons in the spindle are activated, the muscle spindle is stretched, an impulse is sent to the spinal cord, motor neurons that innervate extrafusal fibers are signaled to relax
    d. The muscle spindle is stretched, sensory neurons in the spindle are activated, an impulse is sent to the spinal cord, sensory neurons that innervate intrafusal fibers are signaled to relax

44. After assessing a patient's passive range of motion in the knee, the therapist determines there is limitation in flexion. Which of the following list of structures may be responsible for the restricted range of motion?
    a. Quadriceps, ligaments, knee joint capsule, fascia
    b. Hamstrings, ligaments, knee joint capsule, fascia
    c. Gastrocnemius, ligaments, knee joint capsule, fascia
    d. Ligaments, knee joint capsule, fascia

45. Which of the following lists of joint types is in the correct order for increasing amounts of permitted motion (least mobile to most mobile)?
    a. Hinge, condyloid, saddle
    b. Saddle, hinge, condyloid
    c. Saddle, condyloid, hinge
    d. Hinge, saddle, condyloid

46. Which of the following is NOT a component of a sarcomere?
    a. Actin
    b. D-line
    c. B-Band
    d. I-Band

47. Which of the following correctly lists the structures of a muscle from largest to smallest?
    a. Fasciculus, muscle fiber, actin, myofibril
    b. Muscle fiber, fasciculus, myofibril, actin
    c. Sarcomere, fasciculus, myofibril, myosin
    d. Muscle fiber, myofibril, sarcomere, actin

48. Myosin cross-bridges attach to the actin filament when the sarcoplasmic reticulum is stimulated to release which of the following?
    a. Calcium ions
    b. Acetylcholine
    c. Troponin
    d. Adenosine triphosphate (ATP)

49. Which of the following types of joints are correctly matched with the anatomic joint example given?
    I. Cartilaginous: pubic symphysis
    II. Saddle: thumb carpal metacarpal
    III. Plane: sutures in skull
    IV. Pivot: radial head on ulna

    a. Choices I, II, III
    b. Choices I, II, IV
    c. Choices I, III, IV
    d. All are correct

50. Which of the following upper body movements take place in the sagittal plane?
    I. Elbow extension
    II. Wrist flexion
    III. Shoulder abduction
    IV. Neck left tilt

    a. I and IV
    b. I, III, IV
    c. I and II
    d. II and III

51. What muscle is the primary antagonist in knee flexion?
    a. Hamstrings
    b. Quadriceps
    c. Gastrocnemius
    d. Tibialis anterior

52. What makes bone resistant to shattering?
    a. The calcium salts deposited in the bone
    b. The collagen fibers
    c. The bone marrow and network of blood vessels
    d. The intricate balance of minerals and collagen fibers

53. Using anatomical terms, what is the relationship of the sternum relative to the deltoid?
    a. Medial
    b. Lateral
    c. Superficial
    d. Posterior

English & Language Usage

1. Which sentence below does not contain an error in comma usage for dates?
    a. My niece arrives from Australia on Monday, February 4, 2016.
    b. My cousin's wedding this Saturday June 9, conflicts with my best friend's birthday party.
    c. The project is due on Tuesday, May, 17, 2016.
    d. I can't get a flight home until Thursday September 21.

2. Which of the following sentences uses correct spelling?
    a. Although he believed himself to be a consciensious judge of character, his judgment in this particular situation was grossly erroneous.
    b. Although he believed himself to be a conscientious judge of character, his judgment in this particular situation was grossly erroneous.
    c. Although he believed himself to be a conscientious judge of character, his judgement in this particular situation was grossly erroneous.
    d. Although he believed himself to be a concientious judge of character, his judgemant in this particular situation was grossly erroneous.

3. The stress of preparing for the exam was starting to take its toll on me.

In the preceding sentence, what part of speech is the word *stress*?
    a. Verb
    b. Noun
    c. Adjective
    d. Adverb

4. Select the example that uses the correct plural form.
    a. Rooves
    b. Octopi
    c. Potatos
    d. Fishes

5. Which of these examples uses correct punctuation?
    a. The presenter said, "The award goes to," and my heart skipped a beat.
    b. The presenter said, "The award goes to" and my heart skipped a beat.
    c. The presenter said "The award goes to" and my heart skipped a beat.
    d. The presenter said, "The award goes to", and my heart skipped a beat.

6. Select the sentence in which the word *counter* functions as an adjective.
    a. The kitchen counter was marred and scratched from years of use.
    b. He countered my offer for the car, but it was still much higher than I was prepared to pay.
    c. Her counter argument was very well presented and logically thought out.
    d. Some of the board's proposals ran counter to the administration's policies.

7. In which of the following sentences does the pronoun correctly agree with its antecedent?
    a. Human beings on the planet have the right to his share of clean water, food, and shelter.
    b. Human beings on the planet have the right to their share of clean water, food, and shelter.
    c. Human beings on the planet have the right to its share of clean water, food, and shelter.
    d. Human beings on the planet have the right to her share of clean water, food, and shelter.

8. Every single one of my mother's siblings, their spouses, and their children met in Colorado for a week-long family vacation last summer.

Which of the following is the complete subject of the preceding sentence?
    a. Every single one
    b. Siblings, spouses, children
    c. One
    d. Every single one of my mother's siblings, their spouses, and their children

9. Walking through the heavily wooded park by the river in October, I was amazed at the beautiful colors of the foliage, the bright blue sky, and the crystal-clear water.

Using the context clues in the preceding sentence, which of the following words is the correct meaning of the word foliage?
    a. Leaves of the trees
    b. Feathers of the birds
    c. Tree bark
    d. Rocks on the path

10. Which of the following sentences incorrectly uses italics?
    a. *Old Yeller* is a classic in children's literature, yet very few young people today have read it or even seen the movie.
    b. My favorite musical of all time has to be *The Sound of Music* followed closely by *Les Miserables*.
    c. Langston Hughes's famous poem *Dreams* is the most anthologized of all his works.
    d. When I went to the Louvre, I was surprised at how small Leonardo de Vinci's *Mona Lisa* is compared to other paintings.

11. Which of the following sentences employs correct usage?
    a. It's always a better idea to ask permission first rather than ask for forgiveness later.
    b. Its always a better idea to ask permission first rather than ask for forgiveness later.
    c. It's always a better idea to ask permission first rather then ask for forgiveness later.
    d. Its always a better idea to ask permission first rather then ask for forgiveness later.

12. Which of the following is an imperative sentence?
    a. The state flower of Texas is the blue bonnet.
    b. Do you know if the team is playing in the finals or not?
    c. Take the first right turn, and then go one block west.
    d. We won in overtime!

13. Identify the compound sentence from the following examples:
    a. John and Adam met for coffee before going to class.
    b. As I was leaving, my dad called and needed to talk.
    c. I ran before work and went to the gym afterward for an hour or so.
    d. Felix plays the guitar in my roommate's band, and Alicia is the lead vocalist.

14. Jose had three exams on Monday, so he spent several hours in the library the day before and more time in his dorm room that night studying.

Identify all the words that function as nouns in the preceding sentence:
    a. Jose, exams, hours, library, day, time, room, night
    b. Jose, exams, Monday, hours, library, day, time, room, night
    c. Jose, exams, Monday, he, hours, library, day, time, dorm, night
    d. Exams, Monday, hours, library, day, time, room, night

15. Identify the sentence that uses correct subject-verb agreement.
    a. Each of the students have completed the final project and presentation.
    b. Many players on the basketball team was injured in last night's game.
    c. My friends from school has been trying to talk me in to dance classes.
    d. Everyone in my family has broken a bone except for me.

16. Which of the following sentences has an error in capitalization?
    a. My Mom used to live on the East Coast.
    b. I registered for one semester of Famous Women in Film, but there is not enough room in my schedule.
    c. I prefer traveling on Southwest Airlines because they do not charge baggage fees.
    d. I have never been to Martha's Vineyard or to any other part of New England for that matter.

17. *The exhilarating morning air, combined with the beautiful mountain scenery, inspired me to want to jump right out of bed every morning for a lengthy run.*

From the following words, select one that is used as an adjective in the preceding sentence.
    a. Air
    b. Inspired
    c. Exhilarating
    d. Morning

18. My favorite teacher gave _____ and _____ extra credit on our project.
    a. me, him
    b. he, I
    c. him, I
    d. him, me

19. Which of these sentences uses correct punctuation?
    a. We traveled through six states on our road trip; Texas, New Mexico, Colorado, Wyoming, Utah, and Montana.
    b. We traveled through six states on our road trip: Texas, New Mexico, Colorado, Wyoming, Utah, and Montana.
    c. We traveled through six states on our road trip -- Texas, New Mexico, Colorado, Wyoming, Utah, and Montana.
    d. We traveled through six states on our road trip, Texas, New Mexico, Colorado, Wyoming, Utah, and Montana.

20. Which of the following sentences employs correct usage?
    a. You're going to need to go there to get your backpack from their house.
    b. Your going to need to go there to get you're backpack from their house.
    c. You're going to need to go their to get your backpack from there house.
    d. Your going to need to go their to get you're backpack from there house.

21. Which of the following sentences uses passive voice?
    a. My car was terribly dented by hail during the storm the other night.
    b. My car looked great after the car wash and detailing.
    c. The hail damaged not only my car but the roof of my house as well.
    d. The storm rolled through during the night, taking everyone by surprise.

22. Which of the following sentences correctly uses an apostrophe?
    a. The childrens' choir performed at the Music Hall on Tuesday.
    b. The Smith's went to Colorado with us last summer.
    c. The Joneses' house is currently unoccupied while they are out of the country.
    d. Peoples' attitudes about politics are sometimes apathetic.

23. Which of the following sentences uses incorrect parallel structure?
    a. We worked out every day by swimming, biking, and a run.
    b. The list of craft supplies included scissors, glue, tissue paper, and glitter.
    c. Before I can come over, I need to run to the bank, go to the grocery store, and stop by the dry cleaners.
    d. I love to eat good food, take long walks, and read great books.

24. Which of the following words is spelled incorrectly?
    a. Caffiene
    b. Counterfeit
    c. Sleigh
    d. Receipt

25. Which of these examples shows incorrect use of subject-verb agreement?
    a. Neither of the cars are parked on the street.
    b. Both of my kids are going to camp this summer.
    c. Any of your friends are welcome to join us on the trip in November.
    d. Each of the clothing options is appropriate for the job interview.

26. When it gets warm in the spring, _____ and _____ like to go fishing at Cobbs Creek.

Which of the following word pairs should be used in the blanks above?
    a. me, him
    b. he, I
    c. him, I
    d. he, me

27. Which example shows correct comma usage for dates?
    a. The due date for the final paper in the course is Monday, May 16, 2016.
    b. The due date for the final paper in the course is Monday, May 16 2016.
    c. The due date for the final project in the course is Monday, May, 16, 2016.
    d. The due date for the final project in the course is Monday May 16, 2016.

28. Which of the following uses correct spelling?
    a. Leslie knew that training for the Philadelphia Marathon would take dicsipline and perserverance, but she was up to the challenge.
    b. Leslie knew that training for the Philadelphia Marathon would take discipline and perseverence, but she was up to the challenge.
    c. Leslie knew that training for the Philadelphia Marathon would take disiplin and perservearance, but she was up to the challenge.
    d. Leslie knew that training for the Philadelphia Marathon would take discipline and perseverance, but she was up to the challenge.

Answer Explanations

Reading

1. C: All the details in this paragraph suggest that Brookside is a great place to live, plus the last sentence states that it is an *idyllic neighborhood*, meaning it is perfect, happy, and blissful. Choices *A* and *B* are incorrect, because although they do contain specific details from the paragraph that support the main idea, they are not the main idea. Choice *D* is incorrect because there is no reference in the paragraph to the crime rate in Brookside.

2. B: A passage like this one would likely appear in some sort of community profile, highlighting the benefits of living or working there. Choice *A* is incorrect because nothing in this passage suggests that it is fictional. It reads as non-fiction, if anything. Choice *C* is incorrect because it does not report anything particularly newsworthy, and Choice *D* is incorrect because it has absolutely nothing to do with a movie review.

3. D: In the first sentence, it states very clearly that the Brookside neighborhood is *one of the nation's first planned communities*. This makes it unique, as many other neighborhoods are old, many other neighborhoods exist in Kansas City, and many other neighborhoods have shopping areas. For these reasons, all the other answer choices are incorrect.

4. B: Chapter 4, Section II would have the information for a research paper about how the nation plans to address the problem of child neglect in affected communities. The title of this section is called "Components of the Commission's National Strategy."

5. A: The chapter on page 52 is called "Addressing the Needs of American Indian/Alaska Native Children." Choice *B* is the chapter related to child abuse in disproportionately affected communities. Choice *C* is related to law enforcement and CPS. Choice *D* is related to support for families. Thus, Choice *A* is the correct answer choice.

6. C: Child abuse and neglect is alive and rampant in our communities, and this chapter outlines those who are in dire need of our attention. Choice *A* has more to do with Chapter 2, "Saving Children's Lives Today and Into the Future," and thus is incorrect. Choice *B* relates to Chapter 4, "Reducing Child Abuse and Neglect Deaths in Disproportionately Affected Communities," and is also incorrect. Choice *D* relates to Chapter 7, "Multidisciplinary Support for Families," which is incorrect.

7. B: Choice *B* is correct because a *simile* is a comparison between two unlike things using the words *like* or *as*. Choice *A* is incorrect because *hyperbole* is an exaggeration for affect. Choice *C* is incorrect because *personification* attributes human characteristics to an inanimate object. Choice *D* is incorrect because *alliteration* is a poetic device in which several words begin with the same letter or letters. It is used to add emphasis or affect.

8. A: Choice *A* is correct because there is evidence in the passage to support it, specifically when he mentions catching "a mess of black-fish, which you couldn't buy in New York for a dollar—large fat fellows, with meat on their bones that it takes a pretty long fork to stick through." There is no evidence to support the other answer choices.

9. B: Prodigious means *great in extent, size, or degree*. In this passage, Whitman is comparing the easternmost part of Long Island to a very large alligator. Therefore, the other answer choices are incorrect.

10. C: Choice *C* is correct because it states the fact that education has a positive impact on lowering crime rates, and it tells your reader what you will cover in that paragraph without providing specific details yet. That's what the remainder of the paragraph is for. Choice *A* is incorrect because the paragraph is about the verification of crime statistics. Choice *B* is incorrect because it is a broad generalization that is simply not true. Choice *D*, while it is on topic, is too specific to be a topic sentence but would be an excellent supporting detail.

11. C: This sentence would not be a good thesis statement because it conveys one very specific detail. All the other answer choices would be good thesis statements because they are general enough for an entire essay but specific enough so that the reader knows exactly what the essay will cover.

12. B: The author clearly states that education is crucial to the survival of the human race, and it can be easily inferred that if this is true, then improvements to our educational system are certainly worth fighting for. Choices *A* and *C* are incorrect because there is nothing in the passage that relates to these statements. Choice *D* is incorrect because it directly contradicts what the author states about all children's ability to learn.

13. A: Clearly, this author feels passionately about the importance of education. This is evident especially in the word choices. For this reason, all the other answer choices are incorrect.

14. C: Based on the author's passionate stance about the importance of education for all children, this answer choice makes the most sense. For this reason, all the other answer choices are incorrect.

15. D: The author mentions the importance of parent involvement and communication between school and home. He also devotes one full paragraph to the impact of technology on education. Nowhere in the passage does the author mention the cost of textbooks, so Choice *D* is correct.

16. C: In 1964, the Democratic candidate won 486 electoral votes while the Republican candidate only won 52, and in 1984, almost the complete opposite was true—the Republican candidate won 525 electoral votes, while the Democratic candidate only won 13. Clearly, this was an almost total swing from one party to the other. Choices *A* and *B* are incorrect because the voter turnout, as indicated by the popular vote numbers, did not remain the same or decrease over this twenty-year period. The popular vote turnout increased by approximately twenty thousand over this twenty-year period. Choice *D* is incorrect because the electoral votes won by each party did change during this twenty-year period.

17. A: The Democratic candidate did win the popular vote, but he lost the electoral votes by five, and a closer look at the map reveals that he only won 21 out of the possible 50 states. All the other statements are correct.

18. B: Primary sources are original, first-hand accounts of events or time-periods as they are happening or very close to the time they occurred. Diary entries are excellent primary sources, as are newspaper articles, works of art and literature, interviews, and live recordings. Choice *A* is incorrect because a Wikipedia article is not a reliable source due to the fact that multiple authors can access and manipulate the information. Choices *C* and *D* are incorrect because they are examples of secondary sources. While they might be very reliable and useful, they are not primary sources.

19. C: Italics are often used to indicate emphasis. Choice *A* is incorrect because quotation marks, not italics, are used to indicate dialogue. Choice *B* is incorrect because although italics can also indicate someone's interior thoughts, in this case, it would not make sense for the word *any* to be a thought rather than spoken aloud. Choice *D* is incorrect because volume is typically indicated by capital letters.

20. D: The abbreviation *i.e.* stands for the Latin phrase, "id est" meaning "that is." It is used to clarify an idea, in this case, the term "mollusk." Choice *A* is incorrect because the abbreviation meaning "for example" is *e.g.* Choices *B* and *C* are incorrect because there are no abbreviations in English for these two phrases.

21. D: *Enterprise* most closely means *cause.* Choices *A, B,* and *C* are all related to the term *enterprise.* However, Dickens speaks of a *cause* here, not a company, courage, or a game. *He will stand by such an enterprise* is a call to stand by a cause to enable the working man to have a certain autonomy over his own economic standing. The very first paragraph ends with the statement that the working man *shall . . . have a share in the management of an institution which is designed for his benefit.*

22. B: The speaker's salutation is one from an entertainer to his audience and uses the friendly language to connect to his audience before a serious speech. Recall in the first paragraph that the speaker is there to "accompany [the audience] . . . through one of my little Christmas books," making him an author there to entertain the crowd with his own writing. The speech preceding the reading is the passage itself, and, as the tone indicates, a serious speech addressing the "working man." Although the passage speaks of employers and employees, the speaker himself is not an employer of the audience, so Choice *A* is incorrect. Choice *C* is also incorrect, as the salutation is not used ironically, but sincerely, as the speech addresses the wellbeing of the crowd. Choice *D* is incorrect because the speech is not given by a politician, but by a writer.

23. B: For the working man to have a say in his institution which is designed for his benefit. Choice *A* is incorrect because that is the speaker's *first* desire, not his second. Choices *C* and *D* are tricky because the language of both of these is mentioned after the word *second.* However, the speaker doesn't get to the second wish until the next sentence. Choices *C* and *D* are merely prepositions preparing for the statement of the main clause, Choice *B.*

24. D: Fungi. Choice *A* (the sun) is not even a living thing. Grass (*B*) is a producer, and the frog (*C*) is a consumer. The fungi break down dead organisms and are the only decomposer shown.

25. B: Grasshopper. An herbivore is an organism that eats only plants, and that's the grasshopper's niche in this particular food chain. Grass (*A*) is a producer, the frog (*C*) is a consumer, and the fungi (*D*) is a decomposer.

26. B: While lacrosse does develop some similar skill sets as basketball, it does not belong in an encyclopedia entry about basketball. All the other answer choices do contain relevant information that would likely appear in an encyclopedia entry under "Basketball."

27. C: The word *revere* would not be an entry on this page because the letters *rever* would come after *revea* in alphabetical order. All the other answer choices contain letters that would come between receipt and reveal and would therefore appear as entries on this page.

28. B: According to the label, 72 calories out of the total 230 calories come from fat. This is approximately a third of 230, or 33%. Choice *A* is incorrect because 12% is the percentage of the daily value of total fat found in a serving of this product. Choice *C* is incorrect because 5% is the percentage of the daily value of saturated fat found in a serving of this product. Choice *D* is incorrect because 0% represents the number of grams of trans fat found in a serving of this product.

29. A: This is the correct answer because if Alex ate two cups, that would be exactly three full servings, based on the label information that 2/3 cup is one serving size. One serving contains 230 calories, so three servings would be three times that amount, or 690 calories. Choice *B* is incorrect because that reflects the number of calories in one serving. Choice *C* is incorrect because that reflects the number of calories in two servings. Choice *D* is incorrect because that reflects the number of calories from fat in one serving.

30. D: This is the correct answer because this product only contains 160 mg, or 7% of the daily value of sodium, so this item would be perfectly fine for someone on a low sodium diet to consume. Choice *A* is incorrect because the values of vitamins A and C are relatively low, meaning someone should try to consume more of those throughout the day. Choice *B* is incorrect because this item contains 45% of the daily value of iron, so it is a good source of iron. Choice *C* is incorrect because this item is not too high in dietary fiber for someone consuming 2,000 calories a day.

31. B: The correct answer is *personification* because Dickinson gives death characteristics of a human person. In addition, by capitalizing the word, she has made "Death" a proper noun or name. Choice *A* is incorrect because *hyperbole* is an exaggeration for affect. Choice *C* is incorrect because an *allusion* is a brief or indirect reference to a person, place, or thing from history, culture, literature, or politics. Choice *D* is incorrect because *alliteration* is a poetic device in which several words begin with the same letter or letters. It is used to add emphasis or affect.

32. C: This is the correct answer because the slash mark represents the break between the first line of this poem and the second. A slash mark would not be used to indicate any of the other answer choices.

33. A: This is the correct answer because he makes it clear that sometimes conflict must happen, and that it can even be a good thing.

34. C: Analogy is the correct answer because an analogy is a comparison between two seemingly unlike things, used to help clarify meaning. In this case, Jefferson is comparing what it takes to keep the ideal of liberty alive to a tree. Choice *A* is incorrect because *personification* attributes human traits or characteristics to an inanimate object. Choice *B* is incorrect because an *allusion* is a brief or indirect reference to a person, place, or thing from history, culture, literature, or politics. Choice *D* is incorrect because an *idiom* is an expression whose meaning is not to be taken literally.

35. D: This is the correct answer because the "gov" indicates that this is a government website. If you are traveling overseas, the U.S. government would be a reliable and up-to-date source of information, especially in regard to travel safety. While the other websites may contain some helpful information, and may indeed be worth reading, blogs and wikis may not be as reliable.

36. B: Persuasive is the correct answer because the author is clearly trying to convey the point that history education is very important. Choice *A* is incorrect because expository writing is more informational and less emotional. Choice *C* is incorrect because narrative writing involves story telling. Choice *D* is incorrect because this is a piece of prose, not poetry.

37. C: This is the correct answer because boldface type is often used to indicate emphasis.

Choice *A* is incorrect because quotation marks are used to indicate dialogue. Choice *B* is incorrect because volume is typically indicated by the use of capital letters. Choice *D* is incorrect because there is no way to indicate misspelling by altering the text.

38. A: Choice *A* is correct because the letters *abol* fall between the two guidewords in alphabetical order. All the other answer choices are incorrect because they do not fall between the two guidewords in alphabetical order.

39. D: An antonym is a word that means the opposite, so *genuine* is the antonym of *feigned,* which means falsified or pretended. All the other answer choices are synonyms for the word *feigned*.

40. C: This answer choice is correct because *one of the most intelligent* is a matter of opinion, not a quantifiable fact. All the other answer choices are factual statements.

41. A: This answer choice is correct because it is the only statement that is not based on opinion. Nutritionists' belief in one certain diet *might* be a matter of opinion, but the statement that many do believe in the health benefits of this particular diet is a fact.

42. B: Following the steps in order will change the word *carload* into the word *radical*.

43. A: This is the correct answer choice because there is evidence to the contrary that Martin Luther King Jr. refused to believe that mankind would be bound to the darkness of racism.

44. B: This is the correct answer choice because Martin Luther King Jr. is using an analogy, comparing the evil of racism to the darkness one would experience on a starless night. He is also making the point that just as one cannot see in the dark, racism blinds one to the truth.

45. D: This is the correct answer choice because expository writing involves straightforward, factual information and analysis. It is unbiased and does not rely on the writer's personal feelings or opinions. Choice *A* is incorrect because narrative writing tells a story. Choice *B* is incorrect because persuasive writing is intended to change the reader's mind or position on a topic. Choice *C* is incorrect because technical writing attempts to outline a complex object or process.

46. B: This is the correct answer choice because the passage begins by describing Carver's childhood fascination with painting and later returns to this point when it states that at the end of his career "Carver returned to his first love of art." For this reason, all the other answer choices are incorrect.

47. A: This is the correct answer choice because the passage contains a definition of the term, *agricultural monoculture,* which is very similar to this answer.

48. C: This is the correct answer choice because there is ample evidence in the passage that refers to Carver's brilliance and the fact that his discoveries had a far-reaching impact both then and now. There is no evidence in the passage to support any of the other answer choices.

49. A: It introduces certain insects that transition from water to air. Choice *B* is incorrect because although the passage talks about gills, it is not the central idea of the passage. Choices *C* and *D* are incorrect because the passage does not "define" or "invite," but only serves as an introduction to stoneflies, dragonflies, and mayflies and their transition from water to air.

50. C: The act of shedding part or all of the outer shell. Choices *A, B,* and *D* are incorrect.

51. B: The first paragraph serves as a contrast to the second. Notice how the first paragraph goes into detail describing how insects are able to breathe air. The second paragraph acts as a contrast to the first by stating "[i]t is of great interest to find that, nevertheless, a number of insects spend much of their time under water." Watch for transition words such as "nevertheless" to help find what type of passage you're dealing with.

52: C: The stage of preparation in between molting is acted out in the water, while the last stage is in the air. Choices *A, B,* and *D* are all incorrect. *Instars* is the phase between two periods of molting, and the text explains when these transitions occur.

53. C: The author's tone is informative and exhibits interest in the subject of the study. Overall, the author presents us with information on the subject. One moment where personal interest is depicted is when the author states, "It is of great interest to find that, nevertheless, a number of insects spend much of their time under water."

Math

1. A: Figure out which is largest by looking at the first non-zero digits. Choice *B*'s first non-zero digit is in the hundredths place. The other three all have non-zero digits in the tenths place, so it must be *A, C,* or *D*. Of these, *A* has the largest first non-zero digit.

2. C: 40*N* would be 4000% of *N*. It's possible to check that each of the others is actually 40% of *N*.

3. B: Instead of multiplying these out, the product can be estimated by using $18 \times 10 = 180$. The error here should be lower than 15, since it is rounded to the nearest integer, and the numbers add to something less than 30.

4. C: 85% of a number means multiplying that number by 0.85. So, $0.85 \times 20 = \frac{85}{100} \times \frac{20}{1}$, which can be simplified to $\frac{17}{20} \times \frac{20}{1} = 17$.

5. A: To find the fraction of the bill that the first three people pay, the fractions need to be added, which means finding common denominator. The common denominator will be 60. $\frac{1}{5} + \frac{1}{4} + \frac{1}{3} = \frac{12}{60} + \frac{15}{60} + \frac{20}{60} = \frac{47}{60}$. The remainder of the bill is $1 - \frac{47}{60} = \frac{60}{60} - \frac{47}{60} = \frac{13}{60}$.

6. B: 30% is $\frac{3}{10}$. The number itself must be $\frac{10}{3}$ of 6, or $\frac{10}{3} \times 6 = 10 \times 2 = 20$.

7. A: These numbers to improper fractions: $\frac{11}{3} - \frac{9}{5}$. Take 15 as a common denominator: $\frac{11}{3} - \frac{9}{5} = : \frac{55}{15} - \frac{27}{15} = \frac{28}{15} = 1\frac{13}{15}$ (when rewritten to get rid of the partial fraction).

8. B: Dividing by 98 can be approximated by dividing by 100, which would mean shifting the decimal point of the numerator to the left by 2. The result is 4.2 and rounds to 3.

9. B: $4\frac{1}{3} + 3\frac{3}{4} = 4 + 3 + \frac{1}{3} + \frac{3}{4} = 7 + \frac{1}{3} + \frac{3}{4}$. Adding the fractions gives $\frac{1}{3} + \frac{3}{4} = \frac{4}{12} + \frac{9}{12} = \frac{13}{12} = 1 + \frac{1}{12}$. Thus, $7 + \frac{1}{3} + \frac{3}{4} = 7 + 1 + \frac{1}{12} = 8\frac{1}{12}$.

10. C: The average is calculated by adding all six numbers, then dividing by 6. The first five numbers have a sum of 25. If the total divided by 6 is equal to 6, then the total itself must be 36. The sixth number must be $36 - 25 = 11$.

11. B: Multiplying by 10^{-3} means moving the decimal point three places to the left, putting in zeroes as necessary.

12. B: $\frac{5}{2} \div \frac{1}{3} = \frac{5}{2} \times \frac{3}{1} = \frac{15}{2} = 7.5$.

13. A: The total fraction taken up by green and red shirts will be $\frac{1}{3} + \frac{2}{5} = \frac{5}{15} + \frac{6}{15} = \frac{11}{15}$. The remaining fraction is $1 - \frac{11}{15} = \frac{15}{15} - \frac{11}{15} = \frac{4}{15}$.

14. C: If she has used $\frac{1}{3}$ of the paint, she has $\frac{2}{3}$ remaining. $2\frac{1}{2}$ gallons are the same as $\frac{5}{2}$ gallons. The calculation is $\frac{2}{3} \times \frac{5}{2} = \frac{5}{3} = 1\frac{2}{3}$ gallons.

15. B: Each instance of x is replaced with a 2, and each instance of y is replaced with a 3 to get $2^2 - 2 \times 2 \times 3 + 2 \times 3^2 = 4 - 12 + 18 = 10$.

16. A: To expand a squared binomial, it's necessary to use the *First, Inner, Outer, Last Method*. $(2x - 4y)^2 = 2x \times 2x + 2x(-4y) + (-4y)(2x) + (-4y)(-4y) = 4x^2 - 8xy - 8xy + 16y^2 = 4x^2 - 16xy + 16y^2$.

17. A: Robert accomplished his task on Tuesday in $\frac{3}{4}$ the time compared to Monday. He must have worked $\frac{4}{3}$ as fast.

18. B: To be directly proportional means that $y = mx$. If x is changed from 5 to 20, the value of x is multiplied by 4. Applying the same rule to the y-value, also multiply the value of y by 4. Therefore, $y = 12$.

19. A: Each bag contributes $4x + 1$ treats. The total treats will be in the form $4nx + n$ where n is the total number of bags. The total is in the form $60x + 15$, from which it is known $n = 15$.

20. D: Let a be the number of apples and o the number of oranges. Then, the total cost is $2a + 3o = 22$, while it is also known that $a + o = 10$. Using the knowledge of systems of equations, cancel the o variables by multiplying the second equation by -3. This makes the equation $-3a - 3o = -30$. Adding this to the first equation, the o values cancel to get $-a = -8$, which simplifies to $a = 8$.

21. D: Denote the width as w and the length as l. Then, $l = 3w + 5$. The perimeter is $2w + 2l = 90$. Substituting the first expression for l into the second equation yields $2(3w + 5) + 2w = 90$, or $8w = 80$, so $l = 10$. Putting this into the first equation, it yields $l = 3(10) + 5 = 35$.

22. A: Lining up the given scores provides the following list: 60, 75, 80, 85, and one unknown. Because the median needs to be 80, it means 80 must be the middle data point out of these five. Therefore, the unknown data point must be the fourth or fifth data point, meaning it must be greater than or equal to 80. The only answer that fails to meet this condition is 60.

23. B: If 60% of 50 workers are women, then there are 30 women working in the office. If half of them are wearing skirts, then that means 15 women wear skirts. Since none of the men wear skirts, this means there are 15 people wearing skirts.

24. A: Let the unknown score be x. The average will be $\frac{5\times50+4\times70+x}{10} = \frac{530+x}{10} = 55$. Multiply both sides by 10 to get $530 + x = 550$, or $x = 20$.

25. D: For manufacturing costs, there is a linear relationship between the cost to the company and the number produced, with a y-intercept given by the base cost of acquiring the means of production, and a slope given by the cost to produce one unit. In this case, that base cost is $50,000, while the cost per unit is $40. So, $y = 40x + 50,000$.

26. C: A die has an equal chance for each outcome. Since it has six sides, each outcome has a probability of $\frac{1}{6}$. The chance of a 1 or a 2 is therefore $\frac{1}{6} + \frac{1}{6} = \frac{1}{3}$.

27. B: An equilateral triangle has three sides of equal length, so if the total perimeter is 18 feet, each side must be 6 feet long. A square with sides of 6 feet will have an area of $6^2 = 36$ square feet.

28. D: This problem can be solved by using unit conversions. The initial units are miles per minute. The final units need to be feet per second. Converting miles to feet uses the equivalence statement 1 mile=5,280 feet. Converting minutes to seconds uses the equivalence statement 1 minute=60 seconds. Setting up the ratios to convert the units is shown in the following equation: $\frac{72\ miles}{90\ minutes} \times \frac{1\ minute}{60\ seconds} \times \frac{5280\ feet}{1\ mile} = 70.4$ feet per second. The initial units cancel out, and the new, desired units are left.

29. B: The formula can be manipulated by dividing both sides by the length, l, and the width, w. The length and width will cancel on the right, leaving height by itself.

30. D: This problem can be solved by setting up a proportion involving the given information and the unknown value. The proportion is $\frac{21\ pages}{4\ nights} = \frac{140\ pages}{x\ nights}$. Solving the proportion by cross-multiplying, the equation becomes $21x = 4 \times 140$, where $x = 26.67$. Since it is not an exact number of nights, the answer is rounded up to 27 nights. Twenty-six nights would not give Sarah enough time.

31. D: The slope from this equation is 50, and it is interpreted as the cost per gigabyte used. Since the g-value represents number of gigabytes and the equation is set equal to the cost in dollars, the slope relates these two values. For every gigabyte used on the phone, the bill goes up 50 dollars.

32. A: Setting up a proportion is the easiest way to represent this situation. The proportion becomes $\frac{20}{x} = \frac{40}{100}$, where cross-multiplication can be used to solve for x. The answer can also be found by observing the two fractions as equivalent, knowing that twenty is half of forty, and fifty is half of one-hundred.

33. B: The volume of a cube is the length of the side cubed, and 3 inches cubed is 27 in³. Choice A is not the correct answer because that is 2×3 inches. Choice C is not the correct answer because that is 3×3 inches, and Choice D is not the correct answer because there was no operation performed.

34. D: The volume of a cube is the length of the side cubed, and 5 centimeters cubed is 125 cm³. Choice A is not the correct answer because that is 2×5 centimeters. Choice B is not the correct answer because that is 3×5 centimeters. Choice C is not the correct answer because that is 5×10 centimeters.

35. C: The volume of a rectangular prism is $length \times width \times height$, and $2\ inches \times 4\ inches \times 6\ inches\ is\ 48\ in^3$. Choice A is not the correct answer because that is $2\ inches \times 6\ inches$. Choice B is not the correct answer because that is $4\ inches \times 6\ inches$. Choice D is not the correct answer because that is double of all the sides multiplied together.

36. B: The volume of a rectangular prism is the $length \times width \times height$, and $3cm \times 5cm \times 11cm$ is $165\ cm^3$. Choice A is not the correct answer because that is $3cm + 5cm + 11cm$. Choice C is not the correct answer because that is 15^2. Choice D is not the correct answer because that is $3cm \times 5cm \times 10cm$.

Science

1. C: In any system, the total mechanical energy is the sum of the potential energy and the kinetic energy. Either value could be zero, but it still must be included in the total. Choices A and B only give the total potential or kinetic energy, respectively. Choice D gives the difference in the kinetic and potential energy.

2. A: A Lewis Dot diagram shows the alignment of the valence (outer) shell electrons and how readily they can pair or bond with the valence shell electrons of other atoms to form a compound. Choice B is incorrect because the Lewis Dot structure aids in understanding how likely an atom is to bond or not bond with another atom, so the inner shell would add no relevance to understanding this likelihood. The positioning of protons and neutrons concerns the nucleus of the atom, which again would not lend information to the likelihood of bonding.

3. D: The decibel scale is used to measure the intensity of sound waves. The decibel scale is a ratio of a particular sound's intensity to a standard value. Since it is a logarithmic scale, it is measured by a factor of 10. Choice A is the name of the effect experienced by an observer of a moving wave; Choice B is a particle in an atom; and Choice C is a unit for measuring power.

4. A: For charges, *like charges repel* each other and *opposite charges attract* each other. Negatives and positives will attract, while two positive charges or two negative charges will repel each other. Charges have an effect on each other, so Choices C and D are incorrect.

5. C: The mitochondrion is often called the powerhouse of the cell and is one of the most important structures for maintaining regular cell function. It is where aerobic cellular respiration occurs and where most of the cell's ATP is generated. The number of mitochondria in a cell varies greatly from organism to organism and from cell to cell. Cells that require more energy, like muscle cells, have more mitochondria.

6. A: Photosynthesis is the process of converting light energy into chemical energy, which is then stored in sugar and other organic molecules. The photosynthetic process takes place in the thylakoids inside chloroplast in plants. Chlorophyll is a green pigment that lives in the thylakoid membranes and absorbs photons from light.

7. B: Carbohydrates consist of sugars. The simplest sugar molecule is called a monosaccharide and has the molecular formula of CH_2O, or a multiple of that formula. Monosaccharides are important molecules for cellular respiration. Their carbon skeleton can also be used to rebuild new small molecules. Lipids are fats, proteins are formed via amino acids, and nucleic acid is found in DNA and RNA.

8. B: The secondary structure of a protein refers to the folds and coils that are formed by hydrogen bonding between the slightly charged atoms of the polypeptide backbone. The primary structure is the sequence of amino acids, similar to the letters in a long word. The tertiary structure is the overall shape of the molecule that results from the interactions between the side chains that are linked to the polypeptide backbone. The quaternary structure is the complete protein structure that occurs when a protein is made up of two or more polypeptide chains.

9. C: A hypothesis is a statement that makes a prediction between two variables. The two variables here are the amount of poison and how quickly the rat dies. Choice *C* states that the more poison a rat is given, the more quickly it will die, which is a prediction. Choice *A* is incorrect because it's simply an observation. Choice *B* is incorrect because it's a question posed by the observation but makes no predictions. Choice *D* is incorrect because it's simply a fact.

10. B: The independent variable is the variable manipulated and the dependent variable is the result of the changes in the independent variable. Choice *B* is correct because the amount of poison is the variable that is changed, and the speed of rat death is the result of the changes in the amount of poison administered. Choice *A* is incorrect because that answer states the opposite. Choice *C* is false because the scientist isn't attempting to determine whether the rat will die *if* it eats poison; the scientist is testing how quickly the rat will die depending on *how much* poison it eats. Choice *D* is incorrect because the cage isn't manipulated in any way and has nothing to do with the hypothesis.

11. B: Models are representations of concepts that are impossible to experience directly, such as the 3D representation of DNA, so Choice *B* is correct. Choice *A* is incorrect because theories simply explain why things happen. Choice *C* is incorrect because laws describe how things happen. Choice *D* is false because an observation analyzes situations using human senses.

12. A: A control is the component or group of the experimental design that isn't manipulated—it's the standard against which the resultant findings are compared, so Choice *A* is correct. A variable is an element of the experiment that is able to be manipulated, making Choice *B* false. A constant is a condition of the experiment outside of the hypothesis that remains unchanged in order to isolate the changes in the variables; therefore, Choice *C* is incorrect. Choice *D* is false because collected data are simply recordings of the observed phenomena that result from the experiment.

13. C: An inference is a logical prediction of a why an event occurred based on previous experiences or education. The person in this example knows that plants need water to survive; therefore, the prediction that someone forgot to water the plant is a reasonable inference, hence Choice *C* is correct. A classification is the grouping of events or objects into categories, so Choice *A* is false. An observation analyzes situations using human senses, so Choice *B* is false. Choice *D* is incorrect because collecting is the act of gathering data for analysis.

14. C: Conversion within the metric system is as simple as the movement of decimal points. The prefix *kilo-* means "one thousand," or three zeros, so the procedure to convert kilometers to the primary unit (meters) is to move the decimal point three units to the right. To get to centimeters, the decimal point must be moved an additional two places to the right: 0.78 → 78,000. Choice *A* is false because the decimal point has only been moved one place to right. Choice *B* is incorrect because the decimal point is moved two units in the wrong direction. Choice *D* is false because the decimal has only been moved three units to the right. The problem can also be solved by using the following conversion equation:

$$0.78 \text{km} \times \frac{1,000 \text{m}}{1 \text{km}} \times \frac{100 cm}{1 \text{m}} = 78,000 cm$$

15. B: The answer choices for this question are tricky. Converting to kilometers from miles will yield the choice 7.514 when using the conversion 1 mile = 1.609 km. However, because the value in miles is written to three significant figures, the answer choice should also yield a value in three significant figures, making 7.51 km the correct answer. Choices *C* and *D* could seem correct if someone flipped the conversion upside-down—that is, if they divided by 1.609 instead of multiplied by it.

$$4.67 mi \times \frac{1.609 km}{1 mi} = 7.514 \ or \ 7.51$$

16. B: The position of the clavicle relative to the humerus is medial. Anatomical directions are referenced to the midline (medial and lateral); to the center (proximal and distal); to the front and rear (anterior and posterior); toward the head and tail (cephalic and caudal); and to the head and feet (superior and inferior). In anatomical position, the body stands erect with palms facing forward. The clavicle would be clearly medial and superior to the humerus as it is closer to the midline and head.

17. A: The coronal, or frontal, plane is a vertical plane positioned so that it divides the body into front (ventral) and back (dorsal) regions. The plane is positioned so that the face, kneecap, and toes are on the ventral side, and the vertebrae and heel are on the dorsal side. The coronal plane is one of three body planes. The other two are the transverse and sagittal planes. The transverse plane divides the anatomy into upper (cranial or head) and lower (caudal or tail) regions. The sagittal plane runs front/back perpendicular to the frontal plane and divides the anatomy into right and left regions.

18. C: Cartilage adds mechanical support to joints. It provides a flexible cushion that aids in mobility while offering support. The first two choices are switched—it is ligaments that connect bones at joints and tendons that attach skeletal muscles to bones. *D* is incorrect because arteries, not veins, deliver oxygenated blood.

19. B: The dermis is the skin layer that contains nerves, blood vessels, hair follicles, and glands. These structures are called skin appendages. These appendages are scattered throughout the connective tissue (elastin and collagen), and the connective tissue provides support to the outer layer, the epidermis. The epidermal surface is a thin layer (except feet and palms where it is thick) of continually-regenerating cells that don't have a blood supply of their own, which explains why superficial cuts don't bleed. The hypodermis is the subcutaneous layer underneath the dermis, and it is composed primary of fat in order to provide insulation.

20. D: Mechanical digestion is physical digestion of food and tearing it into smaller pieces using force. This occurs in the stomach and mouth. Chemical digestion involves chemically changing the food and breaking it down into small organic compounds that can be utilized by the cell to build molecules. The salivary glands in the mouth secrete amylase that breaks down starch, which begins chemical digestion. The stomach contains enzymes such as pepsinogen/pepsin and gastric lipase, which chemically digest protein and fats, respectively. The small intestine continues to digest protein using the enzymes trypsin and chymotrypsin. It also digests fats with the help of bile from the liver and lipase from the pancreas. These organs act as exocrine glands because they secrete substances through a duct. Carbohydrates are digested in the small intestine with the help of pancreatic amylase, gut bacterial flora and fauna, and brush border enzymes, like lactose. Brush border enzymes are contained in the towel-like microvilli in the small intestine that soak up nutrients.

21. B: The radius and ulna are the bones from the elbow to the wrist, and the humerus is the bone between the elbow and the shoulder. The tibia and fibula are the bones from the knee to the ankle, and the femur is the bone from the knee to the hip. The other choices are bones in the body as well, just not limb bones. The mandible is the jaw, the scapula is the shoulder blade, and the carpal bones are in the wrist.

22. B: In the Haversian system found in compact bone, concentric layers of bone cells are called lamellae. Between the lamellae are lacunae, which are gaps filled with osteocytes. The Haversian canals on the outer regions of the bone contain capillaries and nerve fibers. Spongy (cancellous) bone is on the extremities of long bones, which makes sense because the ends are softer due to the motion at joints (providing flexibility and cushion). The middle of the bone between the two spongy regions is called the diaphysis region. Spongy bone is highly vascular and is the site of red bone marrow (the marrow that makes red blood cells). Long bones, on the other hand, are long, weight-bearing bones like the tibia or femur that contain yellow marrow in adulthood. Trabeculae is a dense, collagenous, rod-shaped tissue that add mechanical support to the spongy regions of bone. Muscular trabeculae can be found in the heart and are similar in that they offer physical reinforcement.

23. A: Carbon dioxide rich blood is delivered and collected in the right atrium and moved to the right ventricle. The tricuspid valve prevents backflow between the two chambers. From there, the pulmonary artery takes blood to the lungs where diffusion causes gas exchange. Then, blood collects in the left atrium and moves to the left ventricle. The mitral valve prevents the backflow of blood from the ventricle to the atrium. Finally, blood is pumped to the body and released in the aorta.

24. B: Smooth, skeletal, and cardiac muscle have defining characteristics, due to their vastly different functions. All have actin and myosin microfilaments that slide past each other to contract.

Skeletal muscles have long fibers made of clearly defined sarcomeres, which make them appear striated. Sarcomeres consist of alternating dark A bands (thick myosin) and light I bands (thin actin). Upon muscle contraction, fibers slide past each. Skeletal muscles are attached to bone via tendons and are responsible for voluntary movement; their contraction brings bones together. They contain multiple nuclei, due to their bundling into fibers.

Cardiac muscles also contain sarcomeres and appear striated but are branched cells with a single nucleus. Branching allows each cell to connect with several others, forming a huge network that has more strength (the whole is greater than the sum of its parts).

Smooth muscles are non-striated and are responsible for involuntary movement (digestion). They do not form cylindrical fibers like skeletal muscles. Their lack of striations is because they have no sarcomeres, and the filaments are randomly arranged.

25. B: The reflex arc is the simplest nerve pathway. The stimulus bypasses the brain, going from sensory receptors through an afferent (incoming) neuron to the spinal cord. It synapses with an efferent (outgoing) neuron in the spinal cord and is transmitted directly to muscle. There is no interneuron involved in a reflex arc. The classic example of a reflex arc is the knee jerk response. Tapping on the patellar tendon of the knee stretches the quadriceps muscle of the thigh, resulting in contraction of the muscle and extension of the knee.

26. B: Proximal tubule → Loop of Henle → Collecting duct is correct. Kidneys filter blood using nephrons that span the outer renal cortex and inner renal medulla. The inner kidneys are composed of the renal pelvis, which collects urine and sends it to the bladder via the ureters. Filtrate first enters the filtering tube of the nephron via the glomerulus, a bundle of capillaries where blood fluid (but not cells) diffuses into the Bowman's capsule, the entryway into the kidney filtration canal. Bowman's capsule collects fluid, but the nephron actually starts filtering blood in the proximal tubule where necessary ions, nutrients, wastes, and (depending on blood osmolarity) water are absorbed or released. Also, blood pH is regulated, here, as the proximal tubule fine-tunes pH by utilizing the blood buffering system, adjusting amounts of hydrogen ions, bicarbonate, and ammonia in the filtrate. Down the loop of Henle in the renal medulla, the filtrate becomes more concentrated as water exits, while on the way back up the loop of Henle, ion concentration is regulated with ion channels. The distal tubule continues to regulate ion and water concentrations, and the collecting duct delivers the filtrate to the renal pelvis.

27. C: The sympathetic nervous system initiates the "fight-or-flight" response and is responsible for body changes that direct all available energy towards survival. Digestion is completely sacrificed so that energy can be averted to increased heart rate and breathing (thus bronchiole dilation). The liver is stimulated to release glycogen (a carbohydrate based starch) to provide available energy. The parasympathetic is the one responsible for stimulating every-day activities like digestion.

28. A: Motor neurons transmit signals from the CNS to effector tissues and organs, such as skeletal muscle and glands. Sensory neurons carry impulses from receptors in the extremities to the CNS. Interneurons relay impulses from neuron to neuron.

29. C: The cerebellum is important for balance and motor coordination. Aside from the brainstem and cerebellum, the outside portion of the brain is the cerebrum, which is the advanced operating system of the brain and is responsible for learning, emotion, memory, perception, and voluntary movement. The amygdala (emotions), language areas, and corpus collosum all exist within the cerebrum.

30. A: The exocrine portion of the pancreas (the majority of it) is an accessory organ to the digestive system (meaning that food never touches it—it is not part of the alimentary canal). It secretes bicarbonate to neutralize stomach acid and enzymes to aid in digestion. It also regulates blood sugar levels through the complementary action of insulin and glucagon that are located in the Islets of Langerhan (endocrine portion). *A* is incorrect because it is not the growth hormone that stimulates insulin secretion, but rather blood sugar levels.

31. D: The lymphatic system is composed of one-way vessels, lymph, and organs and is designed to filter pathogens and debris from the blood, return nutrients that have leaked from the blood, and maintain, and even stimulate, the immune system if necessary. It circulates lymph, a clear fluid filled with blood plasma that has leaked from capillary beds. The lymphatic system delivers lymph, a clear, colorless fluid, to the neck. It has several organs:

- Lymph nodes, which remove debris from lymph and forms lymphocytes
- The thymus, which develops lymphocytes
- The spleen, which removes pathogens from blood and makes lymphocytes
- Tonsils, which collect debris

The lymphatic system also absorbs lipids and fat-soluble vitamins from the gut and returns them to the circulatory system.

32. C: ADH secretion is correct. Antidiuretic hormone controls water reabsorption. In its presence, water is reabsorbed, and urine is more concentrated. When absent, water is excreted, and urine is dilute. It is a regulator of blood volume, not pH. The other choices do affect blood pH.

$$H_2O + CO_2 \leftrightarrow H_2CO_3 \leftrightarrow H^+ + HCO_3^-$$

This chemical reaction can be fine-tuned in order to tweak the pH. It's helpful to notice the hydrogen ion on the product side of the equation. The more hydrogen ions there are, the more acidic the blood is. Carbonic acid, the "middle-man," regulates blood by being a buffer. Exhaling releases carbon dioxide. This pushes the reaction to the left, which will decrease Hydrogen ions and make blood less acidic. Kidney regulation of bicarbonate will also shift the reaction to the left or right, raising or lowering pH as necessary.

Ammonia secreted by the proximal tubule of the nephron also regulates pH, since it will trap hydrogen ions and convert into ammonium ions. Reduced hydrogen ions make blood less acidic.

$$NH_3 + H^+ \leftrightarrow NH_4^+$$

33. D: The gland that regulates blood calcium levels is the parathyroid gland. Humans have four parathyroid glands located by the thyroid on each side of the neck, just below the larynx. Typical with the endocrine system, the parathyroid glands operate via feedback loops. If calcium in the blood is low, the parathyroid glands produce parathyroid hormone, which circulates to the bones and removes calcium. If calcium is high, they turn off parathyroid hormone production.

34. D: The hypothalamus is the link between the nervous and endocrine system. It receives information from the brain and sends signals to the pituitary gland, instructing it to release or inhibit release of hormones. Aside from its endocrine function, it controls body temperature, hunger, sleep, circadian rhythms, and is part of the limbic system.

35. C: When muscles contract, they pull bones together. They cannot push apart though, so they work in antagonistic pairs where they are on opposite sides of the bone.

When the bicep contracts, the arm bends and the tricep is relaxed; on the other hand, when the tricep contracts, the arm opens, and the bicep relaxes.

The quadriceps on the thigh straighten the knee; the hamstrings behind the thigh bend the knee.

The trapezius, rhomboid major, and rhomboid minor are muscles on the upper back that pull the shoulders back. The pectoralis major and minor (pecs) are on the chest and allow movement of the shoulder (throwing, lifting, rotating).

The gluteus maximus is the buttocks muscle and extends to the hip. It is the major of the glutes and is responsible for large movements like jumping. The gluteus medius and minimus stabilize the pelvis. The antagonist muscle to the gluteus maximus is the iliopasoas, the flexor muscles. Therefore, Choice C is incorrect since the glutes are not antagonistic muscles.

36. A: Platelets are the blood components responsible for clotting. There are between 150,000 and 450,000 platelets in healthy blood. When a clot forms, platelets adhere to the injured area of the vessel and promote a molecular cascade that results in adherence of more platelets. Ultimately, the platelet aggregation results in recruitment of a protein called fibrin, which adds structure to the clot. Too many platelets can cause clotting disorders. Not enough leads to bleeding disorders.

37. A: Choice *B* might be an attractive answer choice, but neutrophils are part of the innate immune system and are not considered part of the primary immune response. The first event that happens in a primary immune response is that macrophages ingest pathogens and display their antigens. Then, they secrete interleukin 1 to recruit helper T cells. Once helper T cells are activated, they secrete interleukin 2 to simulate plasma B and killer T cell production. Only then can plasma B make the pathogen specific antibodies.

38. C: The epididymis stores sperm and is a coiled tube located near the testes. The immature sperm that enters the epididymis from the testes migrates through the 20-foot long epididymis tube in about two weeks, where viable sperm are concentrated at the end. The vas deferens is a tube that transports mature sperm from the epididymis to the urethra. Seminal vesicles are pouches attached that add fructose to the ejaculate to provide energy for sperm. The prostate gland excretes fluid that makes up about a third of semen released during ejaculation. The fluid reduces semen viscosity and contains enzymes that aid in sperm functioning; both effects increase sperm motility and ultimate success.

39. C: The female reproductive system is a symphony of different hormones that work together in order to propagate the species. Below, find the function of each one:

Hormone	Source	Action
GnRH	Hypothalamus	Stimulates anterior pituitary to secrete FSH and LH
FSH	Anterior Pituitary	Stimulates ovaries to develop mature follicles (with ova); follicles produce increasingly high levels of estrogen
LH	Anterior Pituitary	Stimulates the release of the ovum by the follicle; follicle then converted into a corpus luteum that secretes progesterone
Estrogen	Ovary (follicle); placenta	Stimulates repair of endometrium of uterus; negative feedback effect inhibits hypothalamus production of GnRH
Progesterone	Ovary (corpus luteum); placenta	Stimulates thickening of and maintains endometrium; negative feedback inhibits pituitary production of LH
Prolactin	Anterior pituitary	Stimulates milk production after childbirth
Oxytocin	Posterior pituitary	Stimulates milk "letdown"
Androgens	Adrenal glands	Stimulates sexual drive
hCG	Embryo (if pregnancy)	Stimulates production of progesterone

40. A: Epithelial cells line cavities and surfaces of body organs and glands, and the three main shapes are squamous, columnar, and cuboidal. Epithelial cells contain no blood vessels, and their functions involve absorption, protection, transport, secretion, and sensing. Simple squamous epithelial are flat cells that are present in lungs and line the heart and vessels. Their flat shape aids in their function, which is diffusion of materials. Simple cuboidal epithelium is found in ducts, and simple columnar epithelium is found in tubes with projections (uterus, villi, bronchi). Any of these types of epithelial cells can be stacked, and then they are called stratified and not simple.

41. C: During muscle contractions, myosin cross-bridges attach via their globular heads to actin, then they swivel, and detach from actin filaments, causing the ends of the sarcomere to be pulled closer together. Choice *A* is incorrect, because it is essentially the opposite of this. Actin (the thin filament) does not attach to myosin (the thick filaments). Choice *B* is incorrect because the action potential is initiated when calcium leaves—rather than enters—the sarcoplasmic reticulum. Choice *D* is incorrect because fibers do not physically shorten. They slide past one another, shortening the distance between the origin and insertion of the muscle.

42. D: Cartilage and synovial fluid are the primary sources of cushioning to joints during impact. The proprioceptive system is responsible for body awareness, coordinated reflexes for balance, and modifying movements based on neural feedback.

43. A: Muscle spindles like in intrafusal muscle fibers, parallel to the direction of the extrafusal fibers. When a muscle is stretched, the embedded spindles are also stretched, activating sensory neurons in the spindles. This activation sends an impulse to the spinal cord, where the sensory neurons synapse with motor neurons. These motor neurons exit the spinal cord and travel back towards the limb, where they innervate with the extrafusal fibers, which receive the message to relax.

44. D: Passive range of motion assesses the non-contractile joint structures, such as ligaments, capsules, and fascia. Active range of motion would also assess the contractile elements (such as muscles and tendons) in addition to the non-contractile elements. Therefore, the specific muscles involved in knee flexion were not applicable to this question.

45. A: All three joint types given are synovial joints, allowing for a fair amount of movement (compared with fibrous and cartilaginous joints). Of the three given, hinge joints, such as the elbow, permit the least motion because they are uniaxial and permit movement in only one plane. Saddle joints and condyloid joints both have reciprocating surfaces that mate with one another and allow a variety of motions in numerous planes, but saddle joints, such as the thumb carpal metacarpal joint, allow more motion than condyloid joints. In saddle joints, two concave surfaces articulate, and in a condyloid joint, such as the wrist, a concave surface articulates with a convex surface, allowing motion in mainly two planes.

46. B: The smallest unit of a muscle fiber, sarcomeres, contain the actin and myosin proteins responsible for the mechanical process of muscle contractions. Located between two Z-lines, the actin and myosin filaments are configured in parallel, end-to-end, along the entire length of the myofibril. The sarcomere consists of four segments: the A-band, H-zone, I-band, and Z-line. The B-band and D-line are fictitious and are not components of a sarcomere.

47. D: Muscle fibers, also called muscle cells (i.e., myocytes), are long, striated, cylindrical cells that are approximately the diameter of a human hair (50 to 100 um), have many nuclei dispersed on the outside of the cell, and are covered by a fibrous membrane called the sarcolemma. Myofibrils, one of the smaller functional units within a myocyte, consist of long, thin (approximately 1/1000 mm) chains proteins. The smallest unit of a muscle fiber, a sarcomere, contains the actin and myosin proteins responsible for the mechanical process of muscle contractions.

48. A: The sarcoplasmic reticulum is a network of tubular channels and vesicles, which together provide structural integrity to the muscle fiber. The sarcoplasmic reticulum also acts as a calcium ion pump, moving Ca^{2+} ions from the sarcoplasm into the muscle fiber when the action potential reaches the cell. The Ca^{2+} binds with troponin, which causes the tropomyosin to move further into the double helix groove, allowing rapid binding of actin and myosin filaments and the power stroke that pulls the actin toward the center of the sarcomere, resulting in a contraction.

49. B: Choices I, II, and IV are correct. Here are the correct matches:

Fibrous: sutures in skull
Plane: intercarpal
Saddle: thumb
Hinge: elbow
Condyloid: wrist
Pivot: radial head on ulna
Cartilaginous: pubic symphysis

50. C: Elbow extension and wrist flexion are movements that both take place in the sagittal plane (the sagittal plane cuts through the anterior and posterior of the body dividing the body into right and left regions). Shoulder abduction and neck left tilt movements both occur in the frontal plane.

51. B: Antagonists are muscles that oppose the action of the agonist (the primary muscle causing a motion). Hamstrings are the primary knee flexors (the agonists), and the quadriceps fire in opposition. The gastrocnemius does cross the knee joint, so it is a knee flexor, although secondary to the hamstrings. Tibialis anterior is on the shin and is involved in dorsiflexion.

52. D: Bony matrix is an intricate lattice of collagen fibers and mineral salts, particularly calcium and phosphorus. The mineral salts are strong but brittle, and the collagen fibers are weak but flexible, so the combination of the two makes bone resistant to shattering and able to withstand the normal forces applied to it.

53. A: The sternum is medial to the deltoid because it is much closer (typically right on) the midline of the body, while the deltoid is lateral at the shoulder cap. Superficial means that a structure is closer to the body surface and posterior means that it falls behind something else. For example, skin is superficial to bone and the kidneys are posterior to the rectus abdominus.

English & Language Usage

1. A: It is necessary to put a comma between the date and the year and between the day of the week and the month. Choice *B* is incorrect because it is missing the comma between the day of the week and the month. Choice *C* is incorrect because it adds an unnecessary comma between the month and date. Choice *D* is missing the necessary comma between day of the week and month.

2. B: *Conscientious* and *judgment* are both spelled correctly in this sentence. These are both considered commonly misspelled words. One or both words are spelled incorrectly in all the other examples.

3. B: In this sentence, the word *stress* is a noun. While the word *stress* can also act as a verb, in this particular case, it functions as a noun as the subject of the sentence. The word *stress* cannot be used as an adjective or adverb, so these answers are also incorrect.

4. B: The correct answer is o*ctopi,* the plural form of the word *octopus*. Choice *A* is the incorrect spelling of the plural of *roof,* which should be *roofs.* Choice *C* is the incorrect spelling of the plural form of the word *potato*, which should be *potatoes.* Choice *D* is the incorrect plural form of the word *fish*, which remains the same in the singular and the plural, *fish.*

5. A: Quotation marks are used to indicate something someone has said. This is a direct quotation that interrupts, or breaks, the sentence in half. A comma is necessary before the quotation and after it, and inside the quotation marks, to set off the quote from the rest of the sentence. Choice *B* is incorrect because there is no comma at the end of the quotation. Choice *C* is incorrect because there is no comma before or after the quotation. Choice *D* is incorrect because the comma at the end of the quotation is placed outside the quotation marks.

6. C: In this sentence, the word *counter* functions as an adjective that modifies the word *argument.* Choice *A* is incorrect because the word *counter* functions as a noun. Choice *B* is incorrect because the word *counter* functions as a verb. Choice *D* is incorrect because the word *counter* functions as an adverb.

7. B: This sentence correctly uses the plural pronoun *their,* which agrees in number with its antecedent, *human beings*. Choice *A* is incorrect because *his* is a singular pronoun and does not agree in number with the antecedent. Choice *C* is incorrect because *its* is a singular pronoun and usually refers to an object. Choice *D* is incorrect because *her* is a singular pronoun and does not agree with the antecedent.

8. D: *Every single one of my mother's siblings, their spouses, and their children* is the complete subject because it includes who or what is doing the action in the sentence as well as the modifiers that go with it. The other answer choices are incorrect because they only include part of the complete subject.

9. A: The word *foliage* is defined as leaves on plants or trees. In this sentence, the meaning can be drawn from the fact that a heavily wooded area in October would be characterized by the beautiful changing colors of the leaves. The other answer choices do not accurately define the word *foliage*, so they are incorrect.

10. C: Choice *C* is the one that incorrectly uses italics; quotation marks should be used for the title of a short work such as a poem, not italics. Choice *A* correctly italicizes the title of a novel. Choice *B* correctly italicizes the title of both musicals, and Choice *D* correctly italicizes the name of a work of art.

11. A: In this sentence, the commonly misused words *it's* and *than* are used correctly. *It's* is a contraction for the pronoun *it* and the verb *is*. The word *than* accurately shows comparison between two things. The other examples all contain some combination of the commonly misused words *then* and *its*. *Then* is an adverb that conveys time, and *its* is a possessive pronoun. Both are incorrectly used in the other examples.

12. C: This example is an imperative sentence because it gives a command and ends with a period. Choice *A* is a declarative sentence that states a fact and ends with a period. Choice *B* is an interrogative sentence that asks a question and ends with a question mark. Choice *D* is an exclamatory sentence that shows strong emotion and ends with an exclamation point.

13. D: This is a compound sentence because it joins two independent clauses, *Felix plays the guitar in my roommate's band* and *Alicia is the lead vocalist*, with a comma and the coordinating conjunction *and*. Choices *A* and *C* are simple sentences, each containing one independent clause with a complete subject and predicate. Choice *A* does contain a compound subject, *John and Adam,* and Choice *C* contains a compound predicate, *ran and went*, but they are still simple sentences that only contain one independent clause. Choice *B* is a complex sentence because it contains one dependent clause, *As I was leaving,* and one independent clause, *my dad called and needed to talk.* This sentence also contains a compound predicate, *called and needed.*

14. B: This answer includes all the words functioning as nouns in the sentence. Choice *A* is incorrect because it does not include the proper noun *Monday*. The word *he* makes Choice *C* incorrect because it is a pronoun. This example also includes the word *dorm*, which can function as a noun, but in this sentence, it functions as an adjective modifying the word *room*. Choice *D* is incorrect because it leaves out the proper noun *Jose*.

15. D: The simple subject of this sentence, *Everyone*, although it names a group, is a singular noun and therefore agrees with the singular verb form *has*. Choice *A* is incorrect because the simple subject *each* does not agree with the plural verb form *have*. In Choice *B*, the plural subject *players* does not agree with the singular verb form *was*. In Choice *C*, the plural subject *friends* does not agree with the singular verb form *has*.

16. A: In this sentence, the word *Mom* should not be capitalized because it is not functioning as a proper noun. If the possessive pronoun *My* was not there, then it would be considered a proper noun and would be capitalized. *East Coast* is correctly capitalized. Choice *B* correctly capitalizes the name of a specific college course, which is considered a proper noun. Choice *C* correctly capitalizes the name of a specific airline, which is a proper noun, and Choice *D* correctly capitalizes the proper nouns *Martha's Vineyard* and *New England*.

17. C: In this sentence, *exhilarating* is functioning as an adjective that modifies the word *morning*, which in turn, modifies the word *air*. The words *air* and *morning* are functioning as nouns, and the word *inspired* is functioning as a verb in this sentence. Other words functioning as adjectives in the sentence include, *beautiful, mountain, every,* and *lengthy.*

18. D: This is the correct answer because the pronouns *him* and *me* are in the objective case. *Him* and *me* are the indirect objects of the verb *gave*. Choice *A* is incorrect because the personal pronoun in this case, *me*, should always go last. Choices *B* and *C* are incorrect because they contain at least one subjective pronoun.

19. B: In this sentence, a colon is correctly used to introduce a series of items. Choice *A* incorrectly uses a semicolon to introduce the series of states. Choice *C* incorrectly uses a dash to introduce the series. Choice *D* is incorrect because it incorrectly uses a comma to introduce the series.

20. A: This sentence uses the correct form of the contraction *you are* as the subject of the sentence, and it uses the correct form of the possessive pronoun *your* to indicate ownership of the backpack. It also uses the correct form of the adverb *there*, indicating place and the possessive pronoun *their* indicating ownership. Choice *B* is incorrect because it reverses the possessive pronoun *your* and the contraction *you are*. Choice *C* is incorrect because it reverses the adverb *there* and the possessive pronoun *their*. Choice *D* is incorrect because it reverses the contraction *you are* and the possessive pronoun *your* and the possessive pronoun *their* and the adverb *there*.

21. A: In this sentence, the subject *car* is acted upon, rather than completing the action of the sentence. To put this sentence into active voice, the subject should be the hail. Example: *The hail during the storm the other night terribly dented my car*. All the other sentences use active voice because the subject is completing the action of the sentence.

22. C: This sentence correctly places an apostrophe after the plural proper noun *Joneses* to show possession. When a proper name ends in *s*, it is necessary to add *–es* to make it plural, then an apostrophe to make the plural form possessive. In Choice *A*, to make the word *children* possessive, add an apostrophe and then *-s* since the word *children* is already plural. Choice *B* does not need an apostrophe because *Smiths* is plural, not possessive. Choice *D* incorrectly places an apostrophe after the *–s*. In this case, to make *people* possessive, it is necessary to add an apostrophe and then an *–s* since the word *people* is already plural.

23. A: When parallel structure is used, all parts of the sentence are grammatically consistent. Choice *A* uses incorrect parallel structure because *swimming* and *biking* are gerunds, whereas *a run* is an infinitive, so the structure is grammatically inconsistent. Choices *B*, *C*, and *D* all have lists that are grammatically consistent.

24. A: The correct spelling of this word is *caffeine*. This answer, along with Choices *B* and *C* are exceptions to the rule *i before e, except after c*. Choice *D* follows this rule because the letters *ie* follow the letter *c*, so the correct order would be *ei*.

25. A: Choice *A* uses incorrect subject-verb agreement because the indefinite pronoun *neither* is singular and must use the singular verb form *is*. The pronoun *both* is plural and uses the plural verb form of *are*. The pronoun *any* can be either singular or plural. In this example, it is used as a plural, so the plural verb form *are* is used. The pronoun *each* is singular and uses the singular verb form *is*.

26. B: Choice *B* is correct because the pronouns *he* and *I* are in the subjective case. *He* and *I* are the subjects of the verb *like* in the independent clause of the sentence. Choices *A*, *C*, and *D* are incorrect because they all contain at least one objective pronoun (*me* and *him*). Objective pronouns should not be used as the subject of the sentence, but rather, they should come as an object of a verb. To test for correct pronoun usage, try reading the pronouns as if it were the only pronoun in the sentence. For example, *he* and *me* may appear to be the correct answer choices, but try reading them as the only pronoun.

> He like[s] to go fishing…
> Me like to go fishing…
> When looked at that way, *me* is an obviously incorrect choice.

27. A: It is necessary to put a comma between the date and the year. It is also required to put a comma between the day of the week and the month. Choice *B* is incorrect because it is missing the comma between the day and year. Choice *C* is incorrect because it adds an unnecessary comma between the month and date. Choice *D* is missing the necessary comma between day of the week and the month.

28. D: *Discipline* and *perseverance* are both spelled correctly in Choice *D*. These are both considered commonly misspelled words. One or both words are spelled incorrectly in Choices *A*, *B*, and *C*.

ATI TEAS Practice Test #2

Reading

1. After reading *To Kill a Mockingbird*, Louise has been asked to write an expository piece that explores the life, significant achievements, and societal impact of Harper Lee, the book's author. Which of the following sources would yield the most information about the author?
   a. A dictionary
   b. A newspaper article about the author
   c. A study guide for *To Kill a Mockingbird*
   d. A biographical account

2. Read the following words:

   mixed
   thrown
   are
   grown
   beaten
   jumped

   Analyze the list and determine which word does not belong.
   a. Mixed
   b. Are
   c. Grown
   d. Jumped

3. Read the following list of words:

   formaldehyde
   forward
   foliage
   follicle
   format
   fort

   Which of the following words would not be found in a dictionary between the guide words focus and fortitude?
   a. Formaldehyde
   b. Forward
   c. Format
   d. Fort

4. Asbestos was an *insidious* yet popular product, mass produced for over one hundred years. Due to its durability and fire resistance, it was used in a wide range of products, such as houses, cars, and ships. As with tobacco, evidence was presented early on that asbestos was dangerous and had cumulative adverse effects, but production didn't decline until the 1970s.

A dictionary provides four different definitions for *insidious*. Based on the above passage, which definition would fit best?
   a. Awaiting a chance to trap or ensnare
   b. Damaging or deadly but attractive
   c. Having incremental or gradual build-up of harmful effects
   d. Causing catastrophic harm

5. After applying for a job multiple times, Bob was finally granted an interview. During the interview, he fumbled several questions, mispronounced his potential supervisor's name, and forgot the name of the company. Soon it was clear he knew he wouldn't be working there. At the end of the interview, he stood up and, with *spurious* confidence, shook the interviewer's hand firmly.

Based on the context of the word *spurious*, a good substitution might be:
   a. Extreme
   b. Mild
   c. Fake
   d. Genuine

6. Follow the numbered instructions to transform the starting word into a different word.

   1. Start with the word KAKISTOCRACY.
   2. Replace the first K with the first A.
   3. Change the Y to an I.
   4. Move the last C to the right of the last I.
   5. Add a T between the last A and the last I.
   6. Change the K to R.

What is the new word?
   a. Aristocrat
   b. Artistic
   c. Aristocratic
   d. Artifact

Name brand diaper #1	Name brand diaper #2	U-Save discount diaper	Online diaper
88 diapers for $29.99	30 diapers for $12.00	50 diapers for $13.00	100 diapers for $45.00
$4.00 in tax	$2.00 in tax	$3.00 in tax	No tax

7. Marge, who is a new parent, is trying to find the best deal on diapers. She has priced them from several different locations. Based on the chart above, which product offers the best deal?
   a. Name brand diaper #1
   b. Name brand diaper #2
   c. U-Save discount diaper
   d. Online diaper

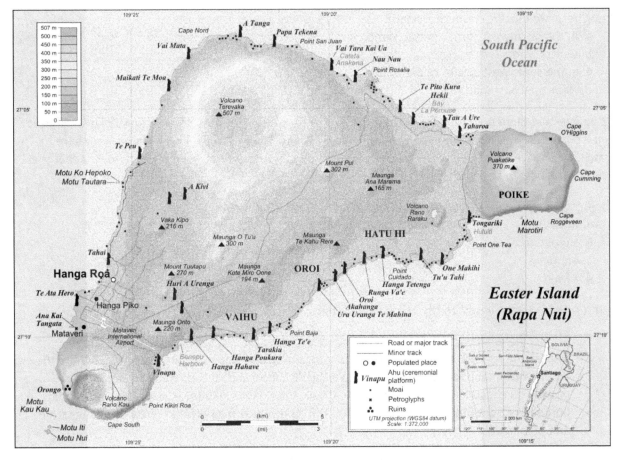

(Eric Gaba, *Wikimedia*, 2016)

Refer to the map above for questions 8–11.

8. How many land masses are represented on this map?
    a. One
    b. Two
    c. Three
    d. Four

9. How many locations are at or above 300 meters?
    a. Four
    b. Five
    c. Six
    d. Seven

10. Where is the most populated area of the island?
    a. In the northwest corner
    b. Centrally located
    c. In the southwest corner
    d. Near the coastline

11. Where are most ruins on the island?
    a. In the northwest corner of the island
    b. Centrally located
    c. In the southwest corner of the island
    d. Near the coastline

12. Reggie had been preparing for his part in the play for several months. His mother had even knitted him a costume. That night when he went on stage, his entire family and all his friends were there to watch, and he was *mortified* when his costume split in half. Afterwards, his mother admitted that she was not the best of seamstresses.

The best substitute for *mortified* would be which of the following?
    a. Inhibited
    b. Humiliated
    c. Annoyed
    d. Afraid

Questions 13–16 are based on the following passage.

Science fiction has been a part of the American fabric for a long time. During the Great Depression, many Americans were looking for an escape from dismal circumstances, and their escape often took the form of reading. Outlandish stories of aliens and superheroes were printed on cheap, disposable paper stock, hence the name *pulp* (as in paper) *fiction*. Iconic heroes like Buck Rogers, the Shadow, and Doc Rogers got their start in throwaway magazines and pulp novels.

As time went on, science fiction evolved, presenting better plots and more sophisticated questions, and, consequently, it garnered more respect. Authors like Kurt Vonnegut and Ray Bradbury, now household names and respected American authors, emerged from the science fiction fringe. Thanks to works like Vonnegut's 1961 short story "Harrison Bergeron," in which mediocrity is the law and exceptional ability is punished, and Bradbury's 1953 novel *Fahrenheit 451*, in which books are illegal and burned on sight, science fiction rose to a serious genre.

In the late 1970s, the genre that begun in the medium of pulp fiction and crossed into serious literature had a resurgence in the medium of film. The new prominence of science fiction film was spearheaded by the first *Star Wars* movie, which harkened to pulp fiction roots. The tide of science fiction films hasn't really slowed since. *Blade Runner*, *Jurassic Park*, *The Matrix*, *I Am Legend*, even Disney's *Wall-E* all continue the tradition of unrealized futures and alternate realities. Modern science fiction movies can trace their roots back to the pulp fiction published during the Great Depression.

13. The main purpose of this passage is to:
    a. Describe
    b. Inform
    c. Persuade
    d. Entertain

14. This passage was written with a _____ structure.
    a. Compare/contrast
    b. Sequential
    c. Cause/effect
    d. Problem/solution

15. Which of the following passages from the above text best summarizes the main idea?
    a. "Science fiction has been a part of the American fabric for a long time."
    b. "As time went on, science fiction evolved, posing better plots and more sophisticated questions."
    c. "Outlandish stories of aliens and superheroes were printed on cheap, disposable paper stock, hence the name *pulp* (as in paper) *fiction*."
    d. "Modern science fiction movies can trace their roots back to the pulp fiction published during the Great Depression."

16. "These outlandish stories of aliens and superheroes were printed on cheap, disposable paper stock, hence the name *pulp* (as in paper) *fiction*." The author most likely wrote this sentence because:
    a. He or she wants the reader to understand that science fiction was not always taken seriously.
    b. He or she wants the reader to understand that science fiction is not a new medium.
    c. He or she wants to demonstrate that science fiction was constrained by the technology of the time.
    d. He or she wants to demonstrate that even those in the past imagined what the future might hold.

Use the following definition to answer questions 17–19.

> A dictionary provides the following information for the word *involve*: in volve (in-volv') v.t. [INVOLVED (-volvd'), INVOLVING], [M.E. *enoulen*; Ofr. *Involver*; L. *involvere*; *in-*, in + *volvere*, to roll up]

17. What does v.t. indicate?
    a. The origin(s) of the word
    b. How to pronounce the word
    c. How to use the word
    d. How many syllables are present

18. What does the space in the word *in volve* indicate?
    a. The origins of the word
    b. How to pronounce the word
    c. How to use the word
    d. How many syllables are present

19. What are the oldest origins for the word *involve*?
    a. Middle English
    b. Old French
    c. Old Germanic
    d. Latin

Use the table below to answer questions 20–23.

	Car 1	Car 2	Car 3	Car 4
Distance Traveled	100 miles	50 miles	70 miles	200 miles
Gallons Needed	4.23 gallons needed	2.083 gallons needed	3.181 gallons needed	8 gallons needed
Size of Tank	12-gallon tank	13-gallon tank	16-gallon tank	14-gallon tank

20. Based on the information above, which car gets the best gas mileage?
    a. Car 1
    b. Car 2
    c. Car 3
    d. Car 4

21. Which car gets the worst gas mileage?
    a. Car 1
    b. Car 2
    c. Car 3
    d. Car 4

22. Which car has the greatest range on one tank of gas?
    a. Car 1
    b. Car 2
    c. Car 3
    d. Car 4

23. Which car has the least range on one tank of gas?
    a. Car 1
    b. Car 2
    c. Car 3
    d. Car 4

Questions 24–27 are based on the following passage.

The more immediately after the commission of a crime a punishment is inflicted, the more just and useful it will be. It will be more just, because it spares the criminal the cruel and superfluous torment of uncertainty, which increases in proportion to the strength of his imagination and the sense of his weakness; and because the privation of liberty, being a punishment, ought to be inflicted before condemnation, but for as short a time as possible. Imprisonments, I say, being only the means of securing the person of the accused, until he be tried, condemned, or acquitted, ought not only to be of as short duration, but attended with as little severity as possible. The time should be determined by the necessary preparation for the trial, and the right of priority in the oldest prisoners. The confinement ought not to be closer than is requisite to prevent his flight, or his concealing the proofs of the crime; and the trial should be conducted with all possible expedition. Can there be a more cruel contrast than that between the indolence of a judge, and the painful anxiety of the accused; the comforts and pleasures of an insensible magistrate, and the filth and misery of the prisoner? In general, as I have before observed, *the degree of the punishment, and the consequences of a crime, ought to be so contrived, as to have the greatest possible effect on others, with the least possible pain to the delinquent.* If there be any society in which this is not a fundamental principle, it is an unlawful society; for mankind, by their union, originally intended to subject themselves to the least evils possible.

An immediate punishment is more useful; because the smaller the interval of time between the punishment and the crime, the stronger and more lasting will be the association of the two ideas of *Crime* and *Punishment;* so that they may be considered, one as the cause, and the other as the unavoidable and necessary effect. It is demonstrated, that the association of ideas is the cement which unites the fabric of the human intellect; without which, pleasure and pain would be simple and ineffectual sensations. The vulgar, that is, all men who have no general ideas or universal principles, act in consequence of the most immediate and familiar associations; but the more remote and complex only present themselves to the minds of those who are passionately attached to a single object, or to those of greater understanding, who have acquired an habit of rapidly comparing together a number of objects, and of forming a conclusion; and the result, that is, the action in consequence, by these means, becomes less dangerous and uncertain.

It is, then, of the greatest importance, that the punishment should succeed the crime as immediately as possible, if we intend, that, in the rude minds of the multitude, the seducing picture of the advantage arising from the crime, should instantly awake the attendant idea of punishment. Delaying the punishment serves only to separate these two ideas; and thus affects the minds of the spectators rather as being a terrible sight than the necessary consequence of a crime; the horror of which should contribute to heighten the idea of the punishment.

There is another excellent method of strengthening this important connexion between the ideas of crime and punishment; that is, to make the punishment as analogous as possible to the nature of the crime; in order that the punishment may lead the mind to consider the crime in a different point of view, from that in which it was placed by the flattering idea of promised advantages.

Crimes of less importance are commonly punished, either in the obscurity of a prison, or the criminal is *transported*, to give, by his slavery, an example to societies which he never offended; an example absolutely useless, because distant from the place where the crime was committed. Men do not, in general, commit great crimes deliberately, but rather in a sudden gust of passion; and they commonly look on the punishment due to a great crime as remote and improbable. The public punishment, therefore, of small crimes will make a greater impression, and, by deterring men from the smaller, will effectually prevent the greater.

(Cesare Beccaria, "Punishments, Advantages of Immediate," *The Criminal Recorder,* 1810).

24. What is the main purpose of this passage?
    a. To describe
    b. To inform
    c. To persuade
    d. To entertain

25. What text structure is this passage using?
    a. Compare/contrast
    b. Sequential
    c. Cause/effect
    d. Problem-solution

26. Which of the following excerpts best exemplifies the main idea of this passage?
    a. "The vulgar, that is, all men who have no general ideas or universal principles, act in consequence of the most immediate and familiar associations."
    b. "Crimes of less importance are commonly punished, either in the obscurity of a prison, or the criminal is *transported*, to give, by his slavery, an example to societies which he never offended."
    c. "Men do not, in general, commit great crimes deliberately, but rather in a sudden gust of passion; and they commonly look on the punishment due to a great crime as remote and improbable."
    d. "The more immediately after the commission of a crime a punishment is inflicted, the more just and useful it will be."

27. With which of the following statements would the author most likely disagree?
    a. Criminals are incapable of connecting crime and punishment.
    b. A punishment should quickly follow the crime.
    c. Most criminals do not think about the consequences of their actions.
    d. Where a criminal is punished is just as important as when.

Cellular Phone 1	Cellular Phone 2	Cellular Phone 3	Cellular Phone 4
Cost of phone: $200	Cost of phone: $100	Cost of phone: $50	Cost of phone: free
Monthly plan: $35	Monthly plan: $25	Monthly plan: $50	Monthly plan: $65
Monthly insurance: $20	Monthly insurance: $30	Monthly insurance: $25	Monthly insurance: $7

28. Taking into consideration the cost of the phone and payments per month, which contract would offer the best value over the course of two months?
    a. Cellular phone 1
    b. Cellular phone 2
    c. Cellular phone 3
    d. Cellular phone 4

29. Taking into consideration the cost of the phone and payments per month, which contract would offer the best value over the course of a year?
    a. Cellular phone 1
    b. Cellular phone 2
    c. Cellular phone 3
    d. Cellular phone 4

30. If someone were accident prone and needed the monthly insurance, which phone would offer the best value over the course of a year?
   a. Cellular phone 1
   b. Cellular phone 2
   c. Cellular phone 3
   d. Cellular phone 4

Questions 31 and 32 are based on the following passage.

Dear Brand-X Employees:

Over the past ten years, Brand-X has been happy to provide free daycare to Brand-X employees. Based on the dedication, long workdays, and professionalism shown daily, it's the least Brand-X management can do. Brand-X wouldn't be where it is today without the hard work of countless, unsung heroes and is truly blessed to have such an amazing staff.

Unfortunately, Brand-X is subject to the same economic forces as any other company. We regret to inform you that, beginning March 15th, Brand-X has decided to discontinue the childcare program. This was a difficult decision to make, one that was arrived at only with the greatest of deliberation. Many other options were discussed, and this seemed to be the only one that allowed Brand-X to still stay competitive while not reducing staff.

Fortunately, all other programs—employee rewards, vacation and sick days, retirement options, volunteer days—have not been impacted. In addition, on Friday we'll be hosting a free lunch buffet. Employees are welcome to wear jeans.

Hope to see you there,

Brand-X Management

31. Which of the following words best describe the tone in the first, second, and third paragraphs?
   a. Relieved; conciliatory; ominous
   b. Conciliatory; ominous; relieved
   c. Proud; apologetic; placating
   d. Placating; apologetic; proud

32. "Unfortunately, Brand-X is subject to the same economic forces as any other company." This line was most likely provided to do what?
   a. Emphasize that Brand-X is no worse than other companies.
   b. Redirect blame from Brand-X to outside forces.
   c. Encourage staff to look for work elsewhere.
   d. Intimidate staff into cooperating.

For his American literature course next fall, Benito's professor submits a required summer reading list to all students. Before the first day of class, Benito is required to read *The Sound and the Fury*, "Barn Burning," *For Whom the Bell Tolls*, *The Grapes of Wrath*, and "A&P."

33. How many books is Benito required to read during the summer?
    a. One
    b. Two
    c. Three
    d. Four

34. How many short stories is Benito required to read during the summer?
    a. One
    b. Two
    c. Three
    d. Four

35. Carl's chore for the day was to clean out a little-used storage shed. When he unlocked the door and walked through it, he got a mouthful of spider web. Brushing his mouth and sputtering, he reached for the light's pull chain. As soon as the bulb went on, a mouse ran between his legs and out the door. *This place is worse than a zoo*, thought Carl as he reached *reluctantly* for a box.

The best replacement for *reluctantly* would be which of the following?
    a. Angrily
    b. Suspiciously
    c. Fearfully
    d. Hesitantly

36. Jason had never been the best student. He had flunked three math tests and turned in only half of his homework. Worrying about his graduation, Jason's mother signed him up for tutoring. Even after several sessions, it was unclear whether he would pass. In the last week of math class, Jason buckled down and passed. Jason's mother marveled at his *gumption*.

The best substitute for *gumption* would be which of the following?
    a. Stubbornness
    b. Laziness
    c. Initiative
    d. Ambition

Questions 37 and 38 are based on the following table.

Ship 1	Ship 2	Ship 3	Ship 4
Depart: 1:10 p.m.	Depart: 1:00 p.m.	Depart: 1:30 p.m.	Depart: 12:30 p.m.
Arrive: 2:30 p.m.	Arrive: 2:45 p.m.	Arrive: 2:20 p.m.	Arrive: 1:50 p.m.
Return: 4:40 p.m.	Return: 5:30 p.m.	Return: 5:30 p.m.	Return: 5:45 p.m.

37. Lucy and Bob both enjoy fishing and want to take a charter ship to an island, but they have different schedules. Lucy, who works mornings, can't leave until 12:45 p.m. She needs thirty minutes to arrive at the dock. Bob, on the other hand, starts work at 6:30 p.m. and needs an hour to get from the docks to his job. There are four different charter ships available. Based on their schedules, which ship would meet both Lucy and Bob's needs?

    a. Ship 1
    b. Ship 2
    c. Ship 3
    d. Ship 4

38. If Lucy and Bob didn't have any time restraints, which boat would give them the most time on the island to fish?

    a. Ship 1
    b. Ship 2
    c. Ship 3
    d. Ship 4

Questions 39–42 are based on the following two passages.

Passage 1

In the modern classroom, cell phones have become indispensable. Cell phones, which are essentially handheld computers, allow students to take notes, connect to the web, perform complex computations, teleconference, and participate in surveys. Most importantly, though, due to their mobility and excellent reception, cell phones are necessary in emergencies. Unlike tablets, laptops, or computers, cell phones are a readily available and free resource—most school district budgets are already strained to begin with—and since today's student is already strongly rooted in technology, when teachers incorporate cell phones, they're "speaking" the student's language, which increases the chance of higher engagement.

Passage 2

As with most forms of technology, there is an appropriate time and place for the use of cell phones. Students are comfortable with cell phones, so it makes sense when teachers allow cell phone use at their discretion. Allowing cell phone use can prove advantageous if done correctly. Unfortunately, if that's not the case—and often it isn't—then a sizable percentage of students pretend to pay attention while *surreptitiously* playing on their phones. This type of disrespectful behavior is often justified by the argument that cell phones are not only a privilege but also a right. Under this logic, confiscating phones is akin to rummaging through students' backpacks. This is in stark contrast to several decades ago when teachers regulated where and when students accessed information.

39. With which of the following statements would both the authors of Passages 1 and 2 agree?
    a. Teachers should incorporate cell phones into curriculum whenever possible.
    b. Cell phones are useful only when an experienced teacher uses them properly.
    c. Cell phones and, moreover, technology, are a strong part of today's culture.
    d. Despite a good lesson plan, cell phone disruptions are impossible to avoid.

40. Which of the following reasons is NOT listed in Passage 1 as a reason for students to have cell phones?
    a. Cell phones are a free, readily available resource.
    b. Cell phones incorporate others forms of technology.
    c. Due to their mobility, cell phones are excellent in an emergency.
    d. Cell phones allow teachers to "speak" clearly with students.

41. Passage 2 includes the statement, "confiscating phones is akin to rummaging through students' backpacks." The author most likely included this statement to do which of the following?
    a. Indicate how unlikely students are to change their minds.
    b. Exemplify how strongly students believe this is a right.
    c. Exemplify how easily the modern student is offended.
    d. Demonstrate how illogical most students' beliefs are.

42. Based on the context of Passage 2, the best substitute for *surreptitiously* would most likely be which of the following?
    a. Privately
    b. Slyly
    c. Obstinately
    d. Defiantly

Questions 43 and 44 are based on the following table.

Cooking Oils	Smoking Point F°	Neutral Taste?
Clarified Butter	485°	No
Peanut Oil	450°	Yes
Lard	374°	No
Safflower Oil	510°	Yes
Coconut Oil	350°	No

43. Zack is getting ready to heat some cooking oil. He knows that if an oil goes above its smoking point, it doesn't taste good. For his recipe, he must get the oil to reach 430° F. Zack has a peanut allergy and would prefer a neutral-tasting oil. Which oil should he use?
    a. Clarified butter
    b. Peanut oil
    c. Safflower oil
    d. Coconut oil

44. If Zack still needed the oil to reach 430° F but he didn't have a peanut allergy and preferred a flavored oil, which oil would he use?
    a. Clarified butter
    b. Peanut oil
    c. Safflower oil
    d. Coconut oil

45. After many failed attempts, Julio made a solemn promise to his mother to clean his room. When she came home from a long day of work, she found her son playing video games, his room still a disaster. Her fists clenched, her eyebrows knitted, she stared down her son and delivered a *vituperative* speech that made him hang his head regretfully.

The best substitute for *vituperative* would be which of the following?
    a. Annoyed
    b. Insult-laden
    c. Passionate
    d. Sorrowful

Questions 46–48 are based on the following passage.

Random Lake Advertisement

Who needs the hassle of traveling far away? This summer, why not rent a house on Random Lake? Located conveniently ten miles away from Random City, Random Lake has everything a family needs. Swimming, kayaking, boating, fishing, volleyball, mini-golf, go-cart track, eagle watching, nature trails—there are enough activities here to keep a family busy for a month, much less a week.

Random Lake hotels are available for every lifestyle and budget. Prefer a pool or free breakfast? Prefer quiet? Historical? Modern? No problem. The Random Lake area has got you covered. House rentals are affordable too. During the summer months, rentals can go as cheaply as 600 dollars a week. Even better deals can be found during the off season. Most homes come fully furnished, and pontoon boats, kayaks, and paddle boats are available for rental. With the Legends and the Broadmoor developments slated for grand openings in March, the choices are endless!

46. The main purpose of this passage is to do what?
    a. Describe
    b. Inform
    c. Persuade
    d. Entertain

47. Which of the following sentences is out of place and should be removed?
    a. "This summer, why not rent a house on Random Lake?"
    b. "There are enough activities here to keep a family busy for a month."
    c. "Pontoon boats, kayaks, and paddle boats are available for rental."
    d. "With several new housing developments slated for grand opening in March, the choices are endless!"

48. Which of the following can be deduced from Passages 1 and 2?
    a. Random City is more populated than Random Lake.
    b. The Random Lake area is newer than Random City.
    c. The Random Lake area is growing.
    d. Random Lake prefers families to couples.

Questions 49–53 are based upon the following passage:

This excerpt is adaptation from "What to the Slave is the Fourth of July?" Rochester, New York, July 5, 1852.

Fellow citizens—Pardon me, and allow me to ask, why am I called upon to speak here today? What have I, or those I represent, to do with your national independence? Are the great principles of political freedom and of natural justice embodied in that Declaration of Independence, Independence extended to us? And am I therefore called upon to bring our humble offering to the national altar, and to confess the benefits, and express devout gratitude for the blessings, resulting from your independence to us?

Would to God, both for your sakes and ours, ours that an affirmative answer could be truthfully returned to these questions! Then would my task be light, and my burden easy and delightful. For who is there so cold that a nation's sympathy could not warm him? Who so obdurate and dead to the claims of gratitude, gratitude that that would not thankfully acknowledge such priceless benefits? Who so stolid and selfish, that would not give his voice to swell the hallelujahs of a nation's jubilee, when the chains of servitude had been torn from his limbs? I am not that man. In a case like that, the dumb may eloquently speak, and the lame man leap as an hart.

But, such is not the state of the case. I say it with a sad sense of the disparity between us. I am not included within the pale of this glorious anniversary. Oh pity! Your high independence only reveals the immeasurable distance between us. The blessings in which you this day rejoice, I do not enjoy in common. The rich inheritance of justice, liberty, prosperity, and independence, bequeathed by your fathers, is shared by *you*, not by *me*. This Fourth of July is *yours,* not *mine.* You may rejoice, *I* must mourn. To drag a man in fetters into the grand illuminated temple of liberty, and call upon him to join you in joyous anthems, were inhuman mockery and sacrilegious irony. Do you mean, citizens, to mock me, by asking me to speak today? If so there is a parallel to your conduct. And let me warn you that it is dangerous to copy the example of a nation whose crimes, towering up to heaven, were thrown down by the breath of the Almighty, burying that nation and irrecoverable ruin! I can today take up the plaintive lament of a peeled and woe-smitten people.

By the rivers of Babylon, there we sat down. Yea! We wept when we remembered Zion. We hanged our harps upon the willows in the midst thereof. For there, they that carried us away captive, required of us a song; and they who wasted us required of us mirth, saying, "Sing us one of the songs of Zion." How can we sing the Lord's song in a strange land? If I forget thee, O Jerusalem, let my right hand forget her cunning. If I do not remember thee, let my tongue cleave to the roof of my mouth.

49. What is the tone of the first paragraph of this passage?
   a. Exasperated
   b. Inclusive
   c. Contemplative
   d. Nonchalant

50. Which word CANNOT be used synonymously with the term *obdurate* as it is conveyed in the text below?

   > Who so obdurate and dead to the claims of gratitude, that would not thankfully acknowledge such priceless benefits?

   a. Steadfast
   b. Stubborn
   c. Contented
   d. Unwavering

51. What is the central purpose of this text?
   a. To demonstrate the author's extensive knowledge of the Bible
   b. To address the feelings of exclusion expressed by African Americans after the establishment of the Fourth of July holiday
   c. To convince wealthy landowners to adopt new holiday rituals
   d. To explain why minorities often relished the notion of segregation in government institutions

52. Which statement serves as evidence of the question above?
   a. By the rivers of Babylon . . . down.
   b. Fellow citizens . . . today.
   c. I can . . . woe-smitten people.
   d. The rich inheritance of justice . . . *not by me.*

53. The statement below features an example of which of the following literary devices?

   > Oh pity! Your high independence only reveals the immeasurable distance between us.

   a. Assonance
   b. Parallelism
   c. Amplification
   d. Hyperbole

Math

1. What is the volume of a cylinder, in terms of π, with a radius of 5 inches and a height of 10 inches?
   a. $250\,\pi$ in^3
   b. $50\,\pi$ in^3
   c. $100\,\pi$ in^3
   d. $200\,\pi$ in^3

2. What is the volume of a cylinder, in terms of π, with a radius of 6 centimeters and a height of 2 centimeters?

    a. $36\,\pi$ cm³

    b. $24\,\pi$ cm³

    c. $72\,\pi$ cm³

    d. $48\,\pi$ cm³

3. What is the volume of a pyramid, with the area of the base measuring 12 inches², and the height measuring 15 inches?

    a. 180 in³

    b. 90 in³

    c. 30 in³

    d. 60 in³

4. What is the volume of a pyramid, with a square base whose side is 6 inches, and the height is 9 inches?

    a. 324 in³

    b. 72 in³

    c. 108 in³

    d. 18 in³

5. What is the volume of a cone, in terms of π, with a radius of 5 inches and height of 9 inches?

    a. $225\,\pi$ in³

    b. $60\,\pi$ in³

    c. $75\,\pi$ in³

    d. $150\,\pi$ in³

6. What is the volume of a cone, in terms of π, with a radius of 10 centimeters and height of 12 centimeters?

    a. 400 cm³

    b. 200 cm³

    c. 120 cm³

    d. 140 cm³

7. What is the volume of a sphere, in terms of π, with a radius of 3 inches?

    a. $36\,\pi$ in³

    b. $27\,\pi$ in³

    c. $9\,\pi$ in³

    d. $72\,\pi$ in³

8. What is the volume of a sphere, in terms of π, with a radius of 6 centimeters?

    a. $144\,\pi$ cm³

    b. $200\,\pi$ cm³

    c. $288\,\pi$ cm³

    d. $120\,\pi$ cm³

9. What is the length of the hypotenuse of a right triangle with one leg equal to 3 centimeters and the other leg equal to 4 centimeters?

  a. 7 cm

  b. 5 cm

  c. 25 cm

  d. 12 cm

10. What is the length of the other leg of a right triangle with a hypotenuse of 10 inches and a leg of 8 inches?

  a. 6 in

  b. 18 in

  c. 80 in

  d. 13 in

11. Using trigonometric ratios for a right angle, what is the value of the angle whose opposite side is equal to 25 centimeters and whose hypotenuse is equal to 50 centimeters?

  a. 15°

  b. 30°

  c. 45°

  d. 90°

12. Using trigonometric ratios for a right angle, what is the value of the closest angle whose adjacent side is equal to 7.071 centimeters and whose hypotenuse is equal to 10 centimeters?

  a. 15°

  b. 30°

  c. 45°

  d. 90°

13. Using trigonometric ratios, what is the value of the other angle whose opposite side is equal to 1 inch and whose adjacent side is equal to the square root of 3 inches?

  a. 15°

  b. 30°

  c. 45°

  d. 90°

14. What is the answer to $(2 + 2i)(2 - 2i)$?

  a. 8

  b. 8i

  c. 4

  d. 4i

15. What is the answer to $(3 + 3i)(3 - 3i)$?

  a. 18

  b. 18i

  c. 9

  d. 9i

16. What is the answer to $\frac{2+2i}{2-2i}$?

    a. 8

    b. 8i

    c. 2i

    d. i

17. What is the answer to $\frac{3+3i}{3-3i}$?

    a. 18

    b. 18i

    c. i

    d. 9i

18. What is 30° converted to radians in terms of π?

    a. $\frac{\pi}{2}$

    b. $\frac{\pi}{3}$

    c. $\frac{\pi}{4}$

    d. $\frac{\pi}{6}$

19. What is 45° converted to radians in terms of π?

    a. $\frac{\pi}{2}$

    b. $\frac{\pi}{3}$

    c. $\frac{\pi}{4}$

    d. $\frac{\pi}{6}$

20. According to building code regulations, the roof of a house has to be set at a minimum angle of 39° up to a maximum angle of 48° to ensure snow and rain will properly slide off it. What is the maximum incline in terms of radians?

    a. $\frac{\pi}{4}$

    b. $\frac{\pi}{15}$

    c. $\frac{4\pi}{15}$

    d. $\frac{3\pi}{4}$

21. An arc is intercepted by a central angle of 240°. What is the number of radians of that angle?

    a. $\frac{3\pi}{4}$

    b. $\frac{4\pi}{3}$

    c. $\frac{\pi}{4}$

    d. $\frac{\pi}{3}$

22. What is $\frac{\pi}{5}$ in terms of degrees?

    a. 10°
    b. 20°
    c. 30°
    d. 36°

23. What is $\frac{\pi}{6}$ in terms of degrees?

    a. 10°
    b. 20°
    c. 30°
    d. 36°

24. The angle of inclination of a ramp is $\frac{\pi}{9}$. What is the measure of that angle in terms of degrees?

    a. 10°
    b. 20°
    c. 25°
    d. 30°

25. A surveyor points her instrument at $\frac{\pi}{18}$. What is the measure of that angle in terms of degrees?

    a. 10°
    b. 20°
    c. 30°
    d. 36°

26. What is the length of an arc, in terms of π, that has an angle of 36° and a circle with a 10 centimeter radius?

    a. $\frac{\pi}{2}$ cm
    b. π cm
    c. 2π cm
    d. 4π cm

27. What is the length of the arc, in terms of π, that has an angle of 72° and a circle with a 20 inch radius?

    a. $8\,\pi$ in
    b. $4\,\pi$ in
    c. $2\,\pi$ in
    d. π in

28. A builder is working with a mason and an architect to create part of a circle for a decorative roof. They need to know the length of the arc, in terms of π, that has an angle of 20° and a circle with a 108 centimeter radius?

    a. $10\,\pi$ cm

    b. $12\,\pi$ cm

    c. $20\,\pi$ cm

    d. $100\,\pi$ cm

29. What is the area of a circle, in terms of π, with a radius of 5 centimeters?

    a. $10\,\pi$ cm ^{2}

    b. $15\,\pi$ cm ^{2}

    c. $20\,\pi$ cm ^{2}

    d. $25\,\pi$ cm ^{2}

30. What is the area of a circle, in terms of π, with a radius of 10 centimeters?

    a. $10\,\pi$ cm ^{2}

    b. $20\,\pi$ cm ^{2}

    c. $100\,\pi$ cm ^{2}

    d. $200\,\pi$ cm ^{2}

31. A pizzeria owner regularly creates jumbo pizzas, each with a radius of 9 inches. She is mathematically inclined and wants to know the area of the pizza in order to purchase the correct boxes and to know how much she is feeding her customers. What is the area of the circle, in terms of π, with a radius of 9 inches?

    a. $81\,\pi$ in ^{2}

    b. $18\,\pi$ in ^{2}

    c. $90\,\pi$ in ^{2}

    d. $9\,\pi$ in ^{2}

32. A landscaper is making a circular garden in his back yard, with a radius of 13 feet. He needs to compute the area to know how much soil to purchase. What is the area of the circle in terms of π?

    a. $26\,\pi$ ft ^{2}

    b. $169\,\pi$ ft ^{2}

    c. $130\,\pi$ ft ^{2}

    d. $260\,\pi$ ft ^{2}

33. What is the length of a chord, whose angle subtended at the center by the chord is 60°, and whose radius is 20 centimeters?

    a. 5 cm

    b. 10 cm

    c. 15 cm

    d. 20 cm

34. What is the length of a chord, whose angle subtended at the center by the chord is 60°, and whose radius is 30 cm?

    a. 5 cm

    b. 10 cm

    c. 15 cm

    d. 20 cm

35. Two chords intersect inside of a circle. The segments of one chord have lengths 3 and $x + 2$. The segments of the other chord have lengths x and $3x + 2$. What are the lengths of these chords?
    a. 1 units
    b. 2 units
    c. 3 units
    d. 6 units

36. Two chords intersect inside of a circle. The segments of one chord have the lengths 4 and $2x + 2$. The segments of the other chord have lengths x and $3x + 2$. What are the lengths of these chords?
    a. 10 units
    b. 2 units
    c. 1 units
    d. 3 units

Science

1. What types of molecules can move through a cell membrane by passive transport?
    a. Complex sugars
    b. Non-lipid soluble molecules
    c. Oxygen
    d. Molecules moving from areas of low concentration to areas of high concentration

2. What is ONE feature that both prokaryotes and eukaryotes have in common?
    a. A plasma membrane
    b. A nucleus enclosed by a membrane
    c. Organelles
    d. A nucleoid

3. What is the LAST phase of mitosis?
    a. Prophase
    b. Telophase
    c. Anaphase
    d. Metaphase

4. How many daughter cells are formed from one parent cell during meiosis?
    a. One
    b. Two
    c. Three
    d. Four

5. What is the name of this compound: CO?
    a. Carbonite oxide
    b. Carbonic dioxide
    c. Carbonic oxide
    d. Carbon monoxide

6. What is the molarity of a solution made by dissolving 4.0 grams of NaCl into enough water to make 120 mL of solution?
    a. 0.34 M
    b. 0.57 M
    c. 0.034 M
    d. 0.057 M

7. Considering a gas in a closed system, at a constant volume, what will happen to the temperature if the pressure is increased?
    a. The temperature will stay the same
    b. The temperature will decrease
    c. The temperature will increase
    d. It cannot be determined with the information given

8. What is the current when a 3.0 V battery is wired across a lightbulb that has a resistance of 6.0 ohms?
    a. 0.5 A
    b. 18.0 A
    c. 0.5 J
    d. 18.0 J

9. Which of the following correctly displays 8,600,000,000,000 in scientific notation (to two significant figures)?
    a. 8.6×10^{12}
    b. 8.6×10^{-12}
    c. 8.6×10^{11}
    d. 8.60×10^{12}

10. The number 0.00067 has how many significant figures?
    a. Six
    b. Five
    c. Three
    d. Two

11. The acceleration of a falling object due to gravity has been proven to be 9.8 m/s^2. A scientist drops a cactus four times and measures the acceleration with an accelerometer and gets the following results: 9.79 m/s^2, 9.81 m/s^2, 9.80 m/s^2, and 9.78 m/s^2. Which of the following accurately describes the measurements?
    a. They're both accurate and precise.
    b. They're accurate but not precise.
    c. They're precise but not accurate.
    d. They're neither accurate nor precise.

12. Which is the correct value for the mean of the following numbers to the appropriate number of significant figures: 3.2, 7.5, 9.6, and 5.4?
    a. 6.4
    b. 6.42
    c. 6.425
    d. 6

13. The following graph demonstrates which type of correlation?

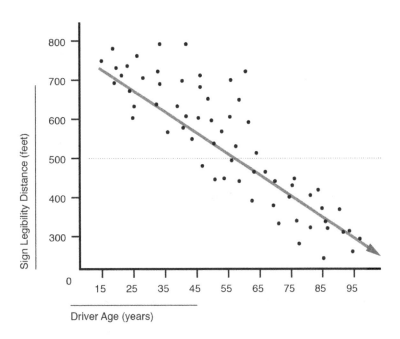

a. Positive correlation
b. No correlation
c. Negative correlation
d. Zero correlation

14. Which of the following is NOT a correct way to handle chemicals or specimens?
a. Always read the safety and data sheets that accompany a product.
b. Don't use substitutions for any chemicals.
c. Keep all work stations clean and sanitized.
d. Always handle chemicals near safety equipment.

15. Which of the following shouldn't be stored in metal?
a. Acids and bases
b. Hydrofluoric gas
c. Gasoline
d. Dihydrogen monoxide

16. Which of the following is NOT a unique property of water?
a. High cohesion and adhesion
b. High surface tension
c. High density upon melting
d. High freezing point

17. What is a metabolic reaction that releases energy called?
a. Catabolic
b. Carbolic
c. Anabolic
d. Endothermic

18. What organic compounds facilitate chemical reactions by lowering activation energy?
    a. Carbohydrates
    b. Lipids
    c. Enzymes
    d. Nucleotides

19. Which structure is exclusively in eukaryotic cells?
    a. Cell wall
    b. Nucleus
    c. Cell membrane
    d. Vacuole

20. Which of these is NOT found in the cell nucleus?
    a. Golgi complex
    b. Chromosomes
    c. Nucleolus
    d. Chromatin

21. What are the energy-generating structures of the cell called?
    a. Nucleoplasms
    b. Mitochondria
    c. Golgi Apparatus
    d. Ribosomes

22. Which is a component of plant cells not found in animal cells?
    a. Nucleus
    b. Plastid
    c. Cell membrane
    d. Cytoplasm

23. Diffusion and osmosis are examples of what type of transport mechanism?
    a. Active
    b. Passive
    c. Extracellular
    d. Intracellular

24. The combination of alleles of an organism, when expressed, manifests as the organism's _____.
    a. genotype.
    b. phenotype.
    c. gender.
    d. karyotype.

25. Which of the choices below are the reproductive cells produced by meiosis?
    a. Genes
    b. Alleles
    c. Chromatids
    d. Gametes

26. What is the process of cell division in somatic (most body) cells called?
    a. Mitosis
    b. Meiosis
    c. Respiration
    d. Cytogenesis

27. When human cells divide by meiosis, how many chromosomes do the resulting cells contain?
    a. 96
    b. 54
    c. 46
    d. 23

28. Which choice is a consequence of tetrad formation in meiosis?
    a. Causes diversity
    b. Determines gender
    c. Causes non-disjunction
    d. Causes transcription

29. What is an alteration in the normal gene sequence called?
    a. DNA mutation
    b. Gene migration
    c. Polygenetic inheritance
    d. Incomplete dominance

30. Blood type is a trait determined by multiple alleles, and two of them are co-dominant: I^A codes for A blood and I^B codes for B blood. i codes for O blood and is recessive to both. If an A heterozygote individual and an O individual have a child, what is the probably that the child will have A blood?
    a. 25%
    b. 50%
    c. 75%
    d. 100%

31. What are the building blocks of DNA referred to as?
    a. Helices
    b. Proteins
    c. Genes
    d. Nucleotides

32. Which statement is NOT true about RNA?
    a. It can be single-stranded.
    b. It has ribose sugar.
    c. It has uracil.
    d. It only exists in three forms.

33. Water has many unique properties due to its unique structure. Which of the following does not play a role in water's unique properties?
    a. Hydrogen bonding between molecules
    b. Polarity within one molecule
    c. Molecules held apart in solid state
    d. Equal sharing of electrons

34. What is the term used for the set of metabolic reactions that convert chemical bonds to energy in the form of ATP?
    a. Photosynthesis
    b. Reproduction
    c. Active transport
    d. Cellular respiration

35. What step happens first in protein synthesis?
    a. mRNA is pulled into the ribosome.
    b. Exons are spliced out of mRNA in processing.
    c. tRNA delivers amino acids.
    d. mRNA makes a complementary DNA copy.

36. What is the idea that evolution involves long periods of stasis and short periods of rapid change?
    a. Natural selection
    b. Punctuated equilibrium
    c. Gradualism
    d. Commensalism

37. Which function below is NOT one of lipids?
    a. Provides cellular instructions
    b. Can be chemical messages
    c. Provides energy
    d. Composes cell membranes

38. What is the cell structure responsible for protein synthesis called?
    a. DNA
    b. Golgi Apparatus
    c. Nucleus
    d. Ribosome

39. Which base pairs with adenine in RNA?
    a. Thymine
    b. Guanine
    c. Cytosine
    d. Uracil

40. With which genotype would the recessive phenotype appear, if the dominant allele is marked with "A" and the recessive allele is marked with "a"?
    a. AA
    b. aa
    c. Aa
    d. aA

41. What is ONE reason why speciation can occur?
    a. Geographic separation
    b. Seasons
    c. Daylight
    d. A virus

42. What is the broadest, or LEAST specialized, classification of the Linnean taxonomic system?
    a. Species
    b. Family
    c. Domain
    d. Phylum

43. How are fungi similar to plants?
    a. They have a cell wall.
    b. They contain chloroplasts.
    c. They perform photosynthesis.
    d. They use carbon dioxide as a source of energy.

44. What important function are the roots of plants responsible for?
    a. Absorbing water from the surrounding environment
    b. Performing photosynthesis
    c. Conducting sugars downward through the leaves
    d. Supporting the plant body

45. Which of the following would occur in response to a change in water concentration?
    a. Phototropism
    b. Thermotropism
    c. Gravitropism
    d. Hydrotropism

46. What is the MAIN function of the respiratory system?
    a. To eliminate waste through the kidneys and bladder
    b. To exchange gas between the air and circulating blood
    c. To transform food and liquids into energy
    d. To excrete waste from the body

47. What type of vessel carries oxygen-rich blood from the heart to other tissues of the body?
    a. Veins
    b. Intestines
    c. Bronchioles
    d. Arteries

48. Which system comprises the 206 bones of the body?
    a. Skeletal
    b. Muscular
    c. Endocrine
    d. Reproductive

49. Which factor is NOT a consideration in population dynamics?
    a. Size and age of population
    b. Immigration
    c. Hair color
    d. Number of births

50. Which type of diagram describes the cycling of energy and nutrients of an ecosystem?
    a. Food web
    b. Phylogenetic tree
    c. Fossil record
    d. Pedigree chart

51. According to Newton's Three Laws of Motion, which of the following is true?
    a. Two objects cannot exert a force on each other without touching.
    b. An object at rest has no inertia.
    c. The weight of an object is the same as the mass of the object.
    d. The weight of an object is equal to the mass of an object multiplied by gravity.

52. What is the chemical reaction when a compound is broken down into its elemental components called?
    a. A synthesis reaction
    b. A decomposition reaction
    c. An organic reaction
    d. An oxidation reaction

53. Which of the following is a balanced chemical equation?
    a. $Na + Cl_2 \rightarrow NaCl$
    b. $2Na + Cl_2 \rightarrow NaCl$
    c. $2Na + Cl_2 \rightarrow 2NaCl$
    d. $2Na + 2Cl_2 \rightarrow 2NaCl$

English & Language Usage

1. Compared to other students, twelve-year-old Dave is somewhat of an oddity at six feet, two inches (tallness runs in his family). The parentheses here indicate what?
    a. The information within is essential to the paragraph.
    b. The information, though relevant, carries less emphasis.
    c. The information is redundant and should be eliminated.
    d. The information belongs elsewhere.

2. The student at a high school, after witnessing some wrongdoing on behalf of others, needed to talk to several _____ based on his _____ .
        a. principals; principles
        b. principles; principals
        c. princapals; princaples
        d. princaples; princapals

3. Each patient, having gone through rehabilitative therapy, needed _____ file returned to the nursing station.
    a. their
    b. there
    c. his or her
    d. the people's

4. A man decided not to take his family to the zoo after hearing about a bomb threat on the news. The man believed the threat to be real and _____ .
   a. eminent
   b. imminent
   c. emanate
   d. amanita

5. Which of the following is punctuated correctly?
   a. Martha expertly read and analyzed a copy of *Taming of the Shrew*: she presented her findings to the class.
   b. Martha expertly read and analyzed a copy of *Taming of the Shrew*, she presented her findings to the class.
   c. Martha expertly read and analyzed a copy of *Taming of the Shrew*; she presented her findings to the class.
   d. Martha expertly read and analyzed a copy of *Taming of the Shrew* she presented her findings to the class.

6. Which of the following exemplifies a compound sentence?
   a. Tod and Elissa went to the movies, got some dessert, and slept.
   b. Though Tod and Elissa decided to go to the movies, Marge stayed home.
   c. Tod and Elissa decided to go to the movies, and Marge read a book.
   d. Tod and Elissa went to the movies while Marge slept.

7. The professor's engaging lecture, though not his best, ran over thirty minutes late. Which of the following words in this preceding sentence functions as a verb?
   a. Engaging
   b. Though
   c. Ran
   d. Over

8. Dave arrived at work almost thirty minutes late. His boss, who was irritated, lectured him. Dave was inconsolable the rest of the shift. Which of the following words in this preceding passage function as an adverb?
   a. Arrived
   b. Almost
   c. Irritated
   d. Rest

9. Which of the following is capitalized correctly?
   a. History 220 is taught by one of my favorite professors. He used to teach an entry-level sociology class but decided he likes teaching Advanced History better.
   b. History 220, taught by Mr. Hart, the Professor, focuses on the conflicts that transformed America: The Revolution, The Civil War, The Korean War, World War I, World War II, and Vietnam.
   c. In particular, he likes to discuss how Yankee ingenuity helped overcome the British army and navy, the world's most formidable world power at the time.
   d. Mr. Hart is scheduled to retire in the summer of 2018. President Williams already said he'll be in charge of retirement party planning.

10. Which of the following passages best displays clarity, fluency, and parallelism?
    a. Ernest Hemingway is probably the most noteworthy of expatriate authors. Hemingway's concise writing style, void of emotion and stream of consciousness, had a lasting impact, one which resonates to this very day. In Hemingway's novels, much like in American cinema, the hero acts without thinking, is living in the moment, and is repressing physical and emotional pain.
    b. Ernest Hemingway is probably the most noteworthy of expatriate authors since his concise writing style is void of emotion and stream of consciousness and has had a lasting impact on Americans which has resonated to this very day, and Hemingway's novels are much like in American cinema. The hero acts. He doesn't think. He lives in the moment. He represses physical and emotional pain.
    c. Ernest Hemingway is probably the most noteworthy of authors. His concise writing style, void of emotion and consciousness, had a lasting impact, one which resonates to this very day. In Hemingway's novels, much like in American cinema, the hero acts without thinking, lives in the moment, and represses physical and emotional pain.
    d. Ernest Hemingway is probably the most noteworthy of expatriate authors. His concise writing style, void of emotion and stream of consciousness, had a lasting impact, one which resonates to this very day. In Hemingway's novels, much like in American cinema, the hero acts without thinking, lives in the moment, and represses physical and emotional pain.

11. Which of the following is punctuated correctly?
    a. After reading *Frankenstein*, Daisy turned to her sister and said, "You told me this book wasn't 'all that bad.' You scare me as much as the book!"
    b. After reading "Frankenstein," Daisy turned to her sister and said, "You told me this book wasn't 'all that bad.' You scare me as much as the book!"
    c. After reading *Frankenstein*, Daisy turned to her sister and said, 'You told me this book wasn't "all that bad." You scare me as much as the book!'
    d. After reading *Frankenstein*, Daisy turned to her sister, and said "You told me this book wasn't 'all that bad'. You scare me as much as the book!"

12. Which of the following subject-verb examples is correct?
    a. Each of the members of the chess club, who have been successful before on their own, struggled to unite as a team.
    b. Everyone who has ever owned a pet and hasn't had help knows it's difficult.
    c. Neither of the boys, after a long day of slumber, have cleaned their bedrooms.
    d. One of the very applauded and commended lecturers are coming to our campus!

13. Sara, who is never late, showed up today ten minutes after Mr. Gray's class had begun. Her hair was a tangled mess, and she looked distraught. Everybody wondered what had happened.

Which of the following words from the preceding passage is an adjective?
    a. Never
    b. After
    c. Mess
    d. Distraught

14. When giving a presentation, one should have three to five bullet points per slide. It is impossible for a presenter to memorize an entire speech, but if you can memorize the main ideas connected to the bullet points, then your speech will be more natural and fluid.

The point(s) of view represented in this passage is/are:
    a. First person only
    b. Third person only
    c. Second person and third person
    d. First person and third person

15. Even though Ralph knew it was wrong to steal, he had still taken a grape from the vegetable stand. He stood there, befuddled, wrestling with his _____ , trying decide whether to put it back or pop it in his mouth.
    a. Conscious
    b. Conscience
    c. Consensus
    d. Census

16. Which of the following demonstrates a simple sentence?
    a. Ted loves to rock climb even though he tore his rotator cuff.
    b. Ted, who is not yet sixty, still easily fishes and camps, too.
    c. Ted loves the outdoors, but, strangely enough, his wife is a homebody.
    d. Ted will also be retired soon; nevertheless, he likes to stay busy.

17. Which of the following examples displays correct use of the possessive?
    a. The womens' portfolios are available for the teacher's review.
    b. A well-trained dog always returns to it's master.
    c. The visitor center is a good place to start the tour.
    d. The businesses' clients had a great time at the convention.

18. An antibiotic is prescribed to eliminate bacterial infections; someone who is antisocial ignores society and laws. Based on these two definitions, the Latin prefix *anti-* would most likely mean:
    a. Reduce
    b. Revolt
    c. Oppose
    d. Without

19. *Conform* means to adjust one's behavior to better fit in with social norms. Inform means to communicate new knowledge to another. Based on these definitions, the Latin suffix *-form* most likely means:
    a. Match
    b. Relay
    c. Negate
    d. Shape

20. Every week, Cindy volunteers time at the local shelter. She always has a smile on her face, and she always talks to others with kindness and patience. Considering that her current job is very taxing, that two of her three children are still in diapers, and that her husband, Steve, the old curmudgeon, is the opposite of her in temperament, it's amazing that no one has ever seen her angry.

Based on the context in this passage, the best substitute for *curmudgeon* would be:
   a. Stingy
   b. Surly
   c. Scared
   d. Shy

21. Most mammals in the New World have prehensile tails while most in Africa do not. Almost all primatologists would agree that animals in places like South America evolved this way to deal with denser vegetation. By moving to a loftier position, animals could avoid predators and move through foliage, unimpeded. On the other hand, it would be less advantageous for a mammal to have a prehensile tail on the African plains. On the long expanses of African savannah, movement is critical for survival, but mammals there would rely on other appendages.

Based on this passage, the best word describing what a *prehensile tail* can do would be:
   a. Grasp
   b. Punch
   c. Move
   d. Walk

22. We went on vacation this summer to Arizona. Mom had always wanted to see the Grand Canyon. Dad, on the other hand, wanted to see Saguaro National Park and Hoover Dam. Other than the flat tire our car got, it was a fantastic time.

The point(s) of view represented in this passage is/are:
   a. First person only
   b. Third person only
   c. Second person and third person
   d. First person and third person

23. Which of the following exemplifies a complex sentence?
   a. To make your fruit last longer, keep it out of the sunlight.
   b. Make sure to clock out after your shift is through.
   c. Making a good fire requires using the proper wood and stacking it properly.
   d. Whenever possible, make sure to yield to oncoming traffic.

24. The people of Scotland are known not only for their unique _____ but also the taxing ____ they make to villages nestled high in the mountains.
   a. Ascents; accents
   b. Accents; ascents
   c. accents; assents
   d. Assents; accents

25. Which of the following sentences has an error in capitalization?
    a. The East Coast has experienced very unpredictable weather this year.
    b. My Uncle owns a home in Florida, where he lives in the winter.
    c. I am taking English Composition II on campus this fall.
    d. There are several nice beaches we can visit on our trip to the Jersey Shore this summer.

26. Julia Robinson, an avid photographer in her spare time, was able to capture stunning shots of the local wildlife on her last business trip to Australia.

Which of the following is an adjective in the preceding sentence?
    a. Time
    b. Capture
    c. Avid
    d. Photographer

27. Which of the following sentences uses correct punctuation?
    a. Carole is not currently working; her focus is on her children at the moment.
    b. Carole is not currently working and her focus is on her children at the moment.
    c. Carole is not currently working, her focus is on her children at the moment.
    d. Carole is not currently working her focus is on her children at the moment.

28. Which of these examples is a compound sentence?
    a. Alex and Shane spent the morning coloring and later took a walk down to the park.
    b. After coloring all morning, Alex and Shane spent the afternoon at the park.
    c. Alex and Shane spent the morning coloring, and then they took a walk down to the park.
    d. After coloring all morning and spending part of the day at the park, Alex and Shane took a nap.

Answer Explanations

Reading

1. D: To find the correct answer, ask what yields the most information and is relevant to the task at hand: finding out about Harper Lee. A dictionary's main purpose is to define words, provide tenses, and establish pronunciation. A newspaper article might offer some information about Harper Lee, but it would be limited in scope to a specific topic or time period. A study guide would focus on literary elements of *To Kill a Mockingbird*, not Harper Lee's life. A biography would be the most comprehensive. It would cover the author, from birth to death, and touch on topics such as upbringing, significant achievements, and societal impacts.

2. B: Unlike all the other words on the list, the word *are* is a being verb. In addition, *are* is in the present tense. The words *mixed, thrown, grown, beaten,* and *jumped* are all action verbs, and they are all in the past tense. The past tense of *are,* of course, is *were.* Therefore, *are* does not fit for two reasons: verb type and tense.

3. B: *Forward* is the correct answer. Since *focus* and *fortitude* are the guide words, all words that fall between them must correspond alphabetically. Formaldehyde, beginning with an f, o, and r, falls after focus, but the next letter, a, places it before fortitude. The f, o, and r in *format* are similar to *formaldehyde,* and, again, the *m* places it before *fortitude.* Lastly, there's *fort.* Since the first four letters match fortitude but there's no additional letters, it would precede fortitude as an entry.

4. C: "Having incremental or gradual build-up of harmful effects" is the correct answer. To find the correct answer, try replacing or substituting words. Here, one might try saying "Damaging or deadly but attractive"; this answer is incorrect because, although the paragraph says the product was popular, it does not indicate that *insidious* means *popular.* "Awaiting a chance to entrap or ensnare" is wrong because asbestos is an inanimate object. "Causing catastrophic harm" doesn't work because the level of harm was not specified in the paragraph.

5. C: To arrive at the correct answer, find the best synonym for *spurious. Fake* makes the most sense because Bob is trying to hide his true emotions. Based on his horrible performance, he understands that he didn't get the job, so the reader can infer that his confidence is not at an all-time high. Therefore, *fake* would make just as much sense in this case as *spurious. Extreme* would indicate that Bob is euphoric and the interview went well. *Mild* would indicate that Bob thought he had a slight chance at getting hired. In this instance, *genuine* would be an antonym; i.e., the exact opposite of what Bob is feeling.

6. C:

> 1. Start with the word KAKISTOCRACY
> 2. Replace the first K with the first A (akistocracy)
> 3. Change the Y to an I. (akistocraci)
> 4. Move the last C to the right of the last I (akistocraic)
> 5. Add a T between the last A and the last I. (akistocratic)
> 6. Change the K to R. (aristocratic)

7. C: U-save discount diaper offers the best deal. To arrive at the correct answer, take the price of the diaper in each column and divide by the number of diapers. Next, take the cost of tax in each column and divide by the numbers of diapers. Add these two totals together to arrive at the total cost per individual diaper. (Note: for the online diaper column, there is no tax to calculate.) The u-save diaper has a total cost of $.26 cents per diaper and $.06 cents tax, totaling $.32 cents per diaper. The first name brand diaper has a cost of $.34 cents per diaper with $.04 cents tax per diaper, totaling $.38 cents per diaper. The second name brand diaper has $.40 cents per diaper and $.06 cents tax per diaper, totaling $.46 cents total per diaper. The online diaper has a cost of $.45 cents per diaper.

8. D: There are four land masses depicted on the map: Easter Island, Motu Kau Kau, Motu Iti, and Motu Nui.

9. A: According to both the number markings and the colored topography, there are four areas above 300 meters: Volcano Terevaka, Volcano Puakatike, Maunga O Tu'u, and Volcano Rano Kau.

10. C: Taking into consideration both the number of roads and the population marker (o) at Hanga Roa, the southwest corner of the island is the most heavily populated.

11. D: Most ruins are located near the coastline, as indicated by the ceremonial platform markers on the key.

12. B: *Humiliated* would be the best substitute for *mortified*. *Inhibited* is a general characteristic of a person unable to act in a relaxed or natural manner; it might be true of Reggie in general but does not describe his acute emotional state at that moment described in the anecdote. *Annoyed* is also too mild a word. *Afraid* is not a synonym of *mortified*.

13. B: The main purpose of this passage was to inform. It wants the reader to understand how American science fiction evolved. Choice A is incorrect because the passage is not very descriptive; there is not an abundance of adjectives and adverbs painting a picture in the reader's mind. The passage is not persuasive (Choice C); the author is not asking the reader to adopt a stance or argument. For Choice D, it might be mildly entertaining, but the entertainment aspect of the passage takes a back seat to its informative aspects.

14. B: This passage begins with the oldest (the pulp fiction magazines of the Great Depression), moves forward to the science fiction of the fifties and sixties via names like Ray Bradbury and Kurt Vonnegut, and ends with a discussion of modern science fiction movies—*Jurassic Park*, *The Matrix*, *I am Legend*. It follows a sequential timeline of American science fiction.

15. A: All other concepts discussed throughout this passage connect to the main idea: "Science fiction has been a part of the American fabric for a long time." Choice B states: "As time went on, science fiction evolved, posing better plots and more sophisticated questions." This is only a portion of the entire history of American science fiction. The same is true of Choice C: "These outlandish stories of aliens and superheroes were printed on cheap, disposable paper stock, hence the name *pulp* (as in paper) *fiction*." Choice D, though it ties together the Great Depression and modern American cinema, doesn't touch on the period in between.

16. A: There are several clues that support Choice A. First, the fact that the stories were printed on *disposable paper* proves that these stories were, at the time, not considered serious literature. Furthermore, it's noted later in the passage that science fiction *was taken seriously* as authors like Kurt Vonnegut and Ray Bradbury gained prominence. This further reinforces the notion that at the beginning it was considered only fanciful and for children. Choice *B* is incorrect. Even though the statement is true of the passage, it's not supported by the individual sentence. Choice *C* is incorrect because the sentence never states directly or hints at this, and, in addition, movies and radio were available during this time period. Choice *D* is incorrect. The premise of the whole passage is that the medium of science fiction is not new. It doesn't spend any time discussing *how* science fiction was written and *what* those authors believed.

17. C: V.t. means the verb is transitive (v.t. is short for the Latin words *verbum transitivum*).

18. D: The hyphen in *involve* is present to indicate how many syllables are present. When people pronounce the word *involve*, there's a break between the *in* and *volve*. The hyphen is there to indicate that break.

19. D: Latin is the oldest origins for the word *involve*. The origins can be traced back through the entry. In Middle English it was *enoulen*; old French used *involver*, and the most ancient version (Latin) is *involvere*.

20. D: Car 4 gets 25 mpg. This is calculated by taking the miles (200) and dividing by the number of gallons needed (8). For car 1, divide 100 by 4.23; it gets 23.6 mpg. For car 2, divide 50 by 2.083; it gets 24 mpg. For car 3, divide 70 by 3.181; it gets 22 mpg. Car 3 gets the worst gas mileage.

21. C: See number 20 above.

22. C: To get the number of miles a car can drive on one tank, multiply the mpg by the size of the tank. For car 1, multiply 23.6 mpg X 12 gallon tank = 283.2 miles. For car 2, 24 mpg X 13 gallon tank = 312 miles. For car 3, 22 mpg X 16 gallon tank = 352 miles. For car 4, 25 mpg X 14 gallon tank = 350 miles. Therefore, car 3 can travel the greatest distance on one tank of gas. Car 1 can travel the least amount with a range of only 283.2 miles.

23. A: See number 22 above.

24. C: Throughout the entire text, the author maintains a persuasive tone. He argues that punishment should quickly follow the crime and gives a host of reasons why: it's more humane; it helps the prisoner to understand the nature of his or her crimes; it makes a better example for society. To confirm it's a persuasive stance, try reversing the argument. If the position cannot be reversed, then it's not persuasive. In this instance, the reader could argue in rebuttal that the punishment does not have to quickly follow the crime. Regardless of the veracity of this argument, simply creating it proves that the passage is persuasive.

25. C: This passage was written with a cause/effect structure. The cause is that the length between incarceration and trial should be as short as possible. The author, then, lists multiple effects of this cause. There are several key words that indicate this is a cause/effect argument. For instance, the author states, "The degree of the punishment, and the consequences of a crime, ought to be so contrived, as to have the greatest possible effect on others, with the least possible pain to the delinquent." The key words *as to have* indicate that changing the manner of punishment will change the outcome. Similarly, the authors states, "An immediate punishment is more useful; because the smaller the interval of time between the punishment and the crime, the stronger and more lasting will be the association of the two ideas of Crime and Punishment." Similar to *as to have* in the previous excerpt, *because* shows causation. In this instance, the author argues that the shorter the duration between crime and punishment, the more criminals will grasp the consequences of their actions. In general, for cause-effect passages, keep a lookout for words like *because, since, consequently, so*, and *as a result*.

26. D: "The more immediately after the commission of a crime a punishment is inflicted, the more just and useful it will be," best exemplifies the main idea of this passage. All subsequent discussion links back to this main idea and plays the role of supporting details. "The vulgar, that is, all men who have no general ideas or universal principles, act in consequence of the most immediate and familiar associations," supports this idea because the "vulgar," criminals, in other words, are used to making quick associations and are not used to delaying gratification or ignoring their impulses. "Crimes of less importance are commonly punished, either in the obscurity of a prison, or the criminal is transported, to give, by his slavery, an example to societies which he never offended," supports the main idea because the author argues that this is the wrong way to punish because if the punishment occurs in the same area the crime was committed, then the punishment will have more effect, since criminals will associate the areas with their crimes. Furthermore, transferring a prisoner takes time and delays punishment. Lastly, the author states, "Men do not, in general, commit great crimes deliberately, but rather in a sudden gust of passion; and they commonly look on the punishment due to a great crime as remote and improbable." To reduce the sense of punishments being remote and improbable, criminals must, according to the author, receive an immediate punishment. Therefore, by removing a lengthy gap between crime and punishment, a criminal's punishment will be close and probable, which the author argues is the most humane way to punish and the mark of a civilized society.

27. A: The author would disagree most strongly with the statement *criminals are incapable of connecting crime and punishment*. Though the author states that criminals are often passionate and consider punishment unlikely in the heat of the crime, the entire premise of the passage is that reducing the time between crime and punishment increases the likelihood of an association. He also argues that if a society does this consistently, the probability that individuals will consider the consequences of their actions increases. *A punishment should quickly follow the crime* is a restatement of the main idea, supported by evidence throughout the passage. *Most criminals do not think about the consequences of their actions*. Though the author makes this clear, he goes on to say that, in general, reducing the time between crime and punishment will have the most positive effect on the prisoner and on society. *Where a criminal is being punished is just as important as when*. The author argues in the passage that a punishment should be immediate and near where the crime originally occurred.

28. D: Cellular phone 4 offers the best value for two months. Since there's no cost for the cell phone, take $65 X 2 = $130. Cellular phone 1: $200 + $35 X 2 = $270. Cellular phone 2: $100 + $25 X 2 = $150. Cellular phone 3: $50 + $45 X 2 = $140.

29. B: Cellular phone 2 offers the best value. Cellular phone 2: $100 + $25 X 12 = $400. Cellular phone 1: $200 + $35 X 12 = $620. Cellular phone 3: $50 + $45 X 12 = $590. Cellular phone 4: $65 X 12 = $744.

30. B: Cellular phone 2 still offers the best value: $100 + ($25 + $30) X 12 = $760. Cellular phone 1: $200 + ($35 + $20) X 12 = $860. Cellular phone 3: $50 + ($45 + $25) X 12 = $890. Cellular phone 4: ($65 + $7) X 12 = $864.

31. C: Brand-X Management uses a proven technique to deliver bad news: sandwich it between good. The first paragraph extolls the virtue of its employees: "Brand-X wouldn't be where it is today without the hard work of countless, unsung heroes and is truly blessed to have such an amazing staff." The management of Brand-X is proud of its employees. The second paragraph delivers the bad news. Along with the announcement of the termination of the childcare program, Brand-X management provides several reasons why, such as they're "subject to the same economic forces as any other company" and their decision "allowed Brand-X to still stay competitive while not reducing staff." The passage implies that they didn't want to—they had to. The tone of the second paragraph is apologetic. The third paragraph ends on a positive note. Management reminds staff that other services—employee rewards, vacation and sick days, retirement options, volunteer days—have not been impacted, and on Friday employees will have a luncheon and be allowed to wear jeans. This passage is there to not only remind employees why it's still beneficial to work there, but also to provide evidence that Brand-X wants its employees to be happy by hosting luncheons and letting employees wear jeans. It's designed to reduce their hostilities about cancelling the program, or, in other words, placate or appease them.

32. B: "Unfortunately, Brand-X is subject to the same economic forces as any other company." This line was most likely provided to redirect blame from Brand-X to outside forces. Throughout the second paragraph, Brand-X consistently defends its decision to cancel the childcare program. Based on the context of the paragraph, it's continually implied that management was left with no choice. While it might be true that Brand-X is no worse than other companies (others are forced to do the same), this statement supports the idea that it's beyond their control, a message reiterated throughout the paragraph. Nowhere in the paragraph does Brand-X encourage employees to look for work elsewhere. In fact, management does the opposite by reminding employees why they want to continue working there: employee rewards, vacation and sick days, retirement options, and volunteer days. The tone of the passage is not intimidating. No threats are made, implied or otherwise. For example, when management makes reference to reducing staff, it's described as an undesirable choice, not a viable option.

33. C: In modern formatting, longer works, such as books, are indicated through the use of italics. Shorter works, such as poems or short stories, are indicated through the use of quotation marks. Accordingly, *The Sound and the Fury*, *For Whom the Bell Tolls*, and *The Grapes of Wrath* are full-length books, while "A&P" and "Barn Burning" are short stories.

34. B: See 33 above.

35. D: Based on what Carl has encountered—a spider web and a mouse—he would be hesitant, lest he encounter another critter. *Fearfully* is too strong a word (unless Carl has a phobia) and would indicate something more serious, like mortal danger. Nowhere in the passage does it indicate Carl is angry, and for Carl to be suspicious, he would have to assume that someone in his life was trying to deceive him. There's no evidence of deception here.

36. C: *Initiative* would be the best replacement for *gumption*. Both words indicate a strong desire to complete a task and overcome obstacles. *Stubbornness* would imply that Jason was resistant to changing his behavior despite it being good or beneficial for him. Despite Jason being lazy, at the end of the passage, he finds the intrinsic motivation necessary to pass the class. The word *ambition* indicates not only a desire for success but also a desire to gain power and influence. Though Jason eventually wants to succeed, he's not trying to gain power or influence.

37. C: To arrive at the correct answer, first calculate the actual times Lucy and Bob could arrive at and depart from the dock. Lucy needs an additional thirty minutes, so that equates to 1:15 p.m., not 12:45. Bob works at 6:30 p.m. and needs an hour subtracted to get to work on time, so that means he would have to leave the dock by 5:30 p.m. Ship 3 leaves at 1:30 p.m., which gives Lucy an additional fifteen minutes' leeway, then returns at 5:30 p.m., which gives Bob the hour he needs to arrive at work on time. Ships 1 and 2 depart at 1:10 p.m. and 1:00 p.m., respectively. Both departure times are too early for Lucy. Ship 4 returns at 5:45 p.m., which is later than Bob can leave the dock for work.

38. D: To arrive at the correct answer, subtract the return times from the arrival times. Assuming it takes approximately the same amount of time for each ship to return, the biggest number should indicate the most amount of time spent on each respective island. Ship 4 provides the most amount of time with 3 hours, 55 minutes. Ship 1 allows 2 hours, 10 minutes; ship 2 is 2 hours, 45 minutes, and ship 3 is 2 hours, 50 minutes.

39. C: Despite the opposite stances in Passages 1 and 2, both authors establish that cell phones are a strong part of culture. In Passage 1 the author states, "Today's student is already strongly rooted in technology." In Passage 2 the author states, "Students are comfortable will cell phones." The author of Passage 2 states that cell phones have a "time and place." The author of Passage 2 would disagree with the statement that *teachers should incorporate cell phones into curriculum whenever possible. Cell phones are useful only when an experienced teacher uses them properly*—this statement is implied in Passage 2, but the author in Passage 1 says cell phones are "indispensable." In other words, no teacher can do without them. *Despite a good lesson plan, cell phone disruptions are impossible to avoid.* This is not supported by either passage. Even though the author in the second passage is more cautionary, the author states, "This can prove advantageous if done correctly." Therefore, there is a possibility that a classroom can run properly with cell phones.

40. D: Here, "speaking" has nothing to do with communication. The original quotation from Passage 1 reads, *Since today's student is already strongly rooted in technology, when teachers incorporate cell phones, they're 'speaking' the student's language.* The first dependent clause makes reference to technology, then uses the word "speaking" as an analogy. The "language" the author refers to is culture. The author never intended the word "speak" to imply actual communication. *Cell phones are a free, readily available resource; cell phones incorporate other forms of technology;* and *due to their mobility, cell phones are excellent in an emergency* are all listed as reasons in Passage 1 to have cell phones.

41. B: The author states in Passage 2, "Confiscating phones is akin to rummaging through students' backpacks." The author most likely included this passage to exemplify how strongly students believe this is a right. This quotation is the evidence or example, and it ties to the previous sentence: "This type of disrespectful behavior is often justified by the argument that cell phones are not only a privilege but also a right." The backpack example illustrates how students believe it's a right. *Indicate how unlikely students are to change their minds; exemplify how easily the modern student is offended* and *demonstrate how illogical most students' beliefs are* are not supported by Passage 2.

42. B: The best substitute for *surreptitiously* would be *slyly.* Let's look at the context of the sentence: "a sizable percentage of a classroom pretends to pay attention while surreptitiously playing on their phones." The key word here is *pretends.* The students in the classroom, therefore, want to use their cell phones but are afraid of getting caught. *Privately* doesn't work because it leaves out the connotation of hiding a wrong act or ulterior motive. *Obstinately* and *defiantly* are also incorrect since students are hiding their disobedience.

43. C: Safflower oil has a smoking point of 510° Fahrenheit. Since Zack's recipe doesn't exceed 430° F, it won't reach the smoking point. In addition, safflower oil doesn't contain peanuts, and safflower oil has a neutral taste. Though clarified butter has a high smoke point, too, it doesn't have a neutral taste. Zack is allergic to peanut oil. Lard, at 374° F, has too low a smoking point and doesn't have a neutral taste. Coconut oil has a smoking point of 350° F and doesn't have a neutral taste.

44. A: Clarified butter has a high smoke point (485°), which would be well above 430° F and doesn't have a neutral taste, which in this scenario Zack prefers. Here, peanut oil is a neutral flavor. Lard, at 374° F, has too low a smoking point. Safflower oil has a smoking point of 510° F, but, here, the flavor is neutral, and he wants a flavored oil. Coconut oil is not neutral, but the smoking point of 350° F is too low.

45. B: *Abusive* would be the best substitute for *vituperative.* Based on the context clues of "long day of work," "fists clenched," and "eyebrows knitted," Julio's mother is angry with her son. Therefore, one can infer that her language will match her nonverbal behavior. *Annoyed* is simply too mild of a word and does not match with her enraged posture. *Passionate* is too vague of a word that can be matched to a different number of moods. *Sorrowful* contradicts the angry posture she's adopted.

46. C: This passage is designed to *persuade*. The whole purpose of the passage is to convince vacationers to come to Random Lake. There are some informative aspects of the passage, such as what's available – boating, house rentals, pontoon boats, but an extremely positive spin is put on the area, a spin that's designed to attract visitors. To prove it's persuasive, the argument can be reversed: Random Lake is *not* a good place to vacation. With a lack of adjectives and adverbs, there's a lack of *descriptive* detail, and this passage doesn't delight or *entertain* like a witty narrative might.

47. C: "Pontoon boats, kayaks, and paddle boats are available for rental" is out of place. The sentence before refers to fully furnished homes, and the sentence after refers to new developments. This sentence would have fit much better near, "Swimming, kayaking, boating, fishing, volleyball, mini-golf, go-cart track, eagle watching, nature trails," because the activities of the area are described. "This summer, why not rent a house on Random Lake?" is followed, logically, by a description of where Random Lake is. "There are enough activities there to keep a family busy for a month," is preceded by a listing of all those activities. "With several new housing developments slated for grand opening in March, the choices are endless!" links to "furnished houses," because this is an opportunity to find even more houses.

48. C: *The Random Lake area is growing.* This can be deduced with the passage, "With the Legends and The Broadmoor developments slated for grand openings in March, the choices are endless!" Considering buildings are being added, not razed, the Random Lake area would have to be growing. *Random City is more populated than Random Lake.* The word *city* is not necessarily indicative of size. There's simply not enough information to determine the size of either Random City or Random Lake. *The Random Lake area is newer than Random City.* Though this might seem logical with the addition of new buildings at Random Lake, there's no way to confirm this. The reader simply doesn't know enough about Random City to draw a comparison. *Random Lake prefers families to couples.* The ad definitely appeals to families but, "There are hotels available for every lifestyle and budget," proves that Random Lake is trying to appeal to everyone. Furthermore, "Prefer quiet? Historical? Modern?" proves that there are accommodations for every lifestyle.

49. A: The tone is exasperated. While contemplative is an option because of the inquisitive nature of the text, Choice *A* is correct because the speaker is annoyed by the thought of being included when he felt that the fellow members of his race were being excluded. The speaker is not nonchalant, nor accepting of the circumstances which he describes.

50. C: Choice *C*, *contented*, is the only word that has a different meaning. Furthermore, the speaker expresses objection and disdain throughout the entire text.

51. B: To address the feelings of exclusion expressed by African Americans after the establishment of the Fourth of July holiday. While the speaker makes biblical references, it is not the main focus of the passage, thus eliminating Choice A as an answer. The passage also makes no mention of wealthy landowners and doesn't speak of any positive response to the historical events, so Choices C and D are not correct.

52. D: Choice D is the correct answer because it clearly makes reference to justice being denied.

53. D: Hyperbole. Choices A and B are unrelated. Assonance is the repetition of sounds and commonly occurs in poetry. Parallelism refers to two statements that correlate in some manner. Choice C is incorrect because amplification normally refers to clarification of meaning by broadening the sentence structure, while hyperbole refers to a phrase or statement that is being exaggerated.

Math

1. A: The volume of a cylinder is $\pi r^2 h$, and $\pi \times 5^2 \times 10$ is $250 \, \pi \, in^3$. Choice B is not the correct answer because that is $5^2 \times 2\pi$. Choice C is not the correct answer since that is $5in \times 10\pi$. Choice D is not the correct answer because that is $10^2 \times 2in$.

2. C: The volume of a cylinder is $\pi r^2 h$, and $\pi \times 6^2 \times 2$ is $72 \, \pi \, cm^3$. Choice A is not the correct answer because that is only $6^2 \times \pi$. Choice B is not the correct answer because that is $2^2 \times 6 \times \pi$. Choice D is not the correct answer because that is $2^3 \times 6 \times \pi$.

3. D: The volume of a pyramid is $(length \times width \times height)$, divided by 3, and (12×15), divided by 3 is 60 in³. Choice A is not the correct answer because that is 12×15. Choice B is not the correct answer because that is (12×15), divided by 2. Choice C is not the correct answer because that is 15×2.

4. C: The volume of a pyramid is $(length \times width \times height)$, divided by 3, and $(6 \times 6 \times 9)$, divided by 3 is 108 in³. Choice A is incorrect because 324 in³ is $(length \times width \times height)$ without dividing by 3. Choice B is incorrect because 6 is used for height instead of 9 [$(6 \times 6 \times 6)$ divided by 3] to get 72 in³. Choice D is incorrect because 18 in³ is (6×9), divided by 3 and leaving out a 6.

5. C: The volume of a cone is $(\pi r^2 h)$, divided by 3, and $(\pi \times 5^2 \times 9)$, divided by 3 is 75 in³. Choice A is not the correct answer because that is $5^2 \times 9$. Choice B is not the correct answer because that is 12×5. Choice D is not the correct answer because that is $5^3 \times 2$.

6. A: The volume of a cone is $(\pi r^2 h)$, divided by 3, and $(\pi \times 10^2 \times 12)$, divided by 3 is 400 cm³. Choice B is $10^2 \times 2$. Choice C is incorrect because it is 10×12. Choice D is also incorrect because that is $10^2 + 40$.

7. A: The formula for the volume of a sphere is $\frac{4}{3}\pi r^3$, and $\frac{4}{3} \times \pi \times 3^3$ is $36 \, \pi \, in^3$. Choice B is not the correct answer because that is only 3^3. Choice C is not the correct answer because that is 3^2, and Choice D is not the correct answer because that is 36×2.

8. C: The formula for the volume of a sphere is $\frac{4}{3}\pi r^3$, and $\frac{4}{3} \times \pi \times 6^3$ is $288 \, \pi \, in^3$. Choice A is not the correct answer because that is 12^2. Choice B is not the correct answer because that is 10^2, and Choice D is not the correct answer because that is $6 \times 2 \times 10$.

9. B: This answer is correct because $3^2 + 4^2$ is $9 + 16$, which is 25. Taking the square root of 25 is 5. Choice A is not the correct answer because that is $3 + 4$. Choice C is not the correct answer because that is stopping at $3^2 + 4^2$ is $9 + 16$, which is 25. Choice D is not the correct answer because that is 3×4.

10. A: This answer is correct because $100 - 64$ is 36 and taking the square root of 36 is 6. Choice B is not the correct answer because that is $10 + 8$. Choice C is not the correct answer because that is 8×10. Choice D is also not the correct answer because there is no reason to arrive at that number.

11. B: The sine of 30° is equal to $\frac{1}{2}$. Choice A is not the correct answer because the sine of 15° is .2588. Choice C is not the answer because the sine of 45° is .707. Choice D is not the answer because the sine of 90 degrees is 1.

12. C: The cosine of 45° is equal to .7071. Choice A is not the correct answer because the cosine of 15° is .9659. Choice B is not the correct answer because the cosine of 30° is .8660. Choice D is not correct because the cosine of 90° is 0.

13. B: The tangent of 30° is 1 over the square root of 3. Choice A is not the correct answer because the tangent of 15° is .2679. Choice C is not the correct answer because the tangent of 45° is 1. Choice D is not the correct answer because the tangent of 90° is undefined.

14. A: This answer is correct because $(2 + 2i)(2 - 2i)$, using the FOIL method is: $4 - 4i + 4i - 4i^2 = 8$. Choice B is not the answer because there is no i in the final answer, since the i's cancel out in the FOIL. Choice C, 4, is not the final answer because we add $4 + 4$ in the end to equal 8. Choice D, 4i, is not the final answer because there is neither a 4 nor an i in the final answer.

15. A: This answer is correct because $(3 + 3i)(3 - 3i)$, using the FOIL method is: $9 - 9i + 9i - 9i2 = 18$. Choice B is not the answer because there is no i in the final answer, since the i's cancel out in the FOIL. Choice C is not the final answer because you have to add the two 9s together in the FOIL method. Choice D is not the final answer because there is neither a 9 nor an i in the final answer.

16. D: Multiply the top and the bottom by $(2 + 2i)$, the conjugate, to arrive at $\frac{8i}{8}$, which cancels to i. Choice A is not the answer because the 8's cancel out. Choice B is not the answer because the 8's cancel out. Choice C is not the answer because 2 is not left, but 8 is.

17. C: First, factor out the 3's: $\frac{1+i}{1-i}$. Then multiply top and bottom by that conjugate: $1 + i \rightarrow \frac{1+2i+i^2}{1-i^2}$. Since i is the square root of -1, this goes to: $\frac{1+2i+(-1)}{1-(-1)}$. This equates to $\frac{2i}{2}$. Cancelling out the 2's leaves i. Choice A is not the correct answer because that only represents the denominator that is part of a fraction that needs to be simplified. Choice B is not the correct answer because that only represents the numerator that is part of a fraction that needs to be simplified. Choice D is not the final answer because it shows only part of the result from the FOIL method.

18. D: When you simplify $\frac{30°\times\pi}{180}$, you get: $\frac{\pi}{6}$. Choice A is not the correct answer because $\frac{\pi}{2} = 90°$. Choice B is not the correct answer because $\frac{\pi}{3} = 60°$. Choice C is not the correct answer because $\frac{\pi}{4} = 45°$.

19. C: When you simplify $\frac{45°\times\pi}{180}$, you get $\frac{\pi}{4}$. Choice A is not the correct answer because $\frac{\pi}{2} = 90°$. Choice B is not the correct answer because $\frac{\pi}{3} = 60°$. Choice D is not the correct answer because $\frac{\pi}{6} = 30°$.

20. C: When you simplify $\frac{48°\times\pi}{180}$, you get $\frac{4\pi}{15}$. Choice A is not the correct answer because $\frac{\pi}{4}$ is 45°. Choice B is not the correct answer because $\frac{\pi}{15}$ is 12°. Choice D is not the correct answer because $\frac{3\pi}{4} = 135°$.

21. B: When you simplify $(\frac{4\pi}{3}) \times (\frac{\pi}{180})$, you get $\frac{4\pi}{3}$. Choice A is not the correct answer because it is the reciprocal of $\frac{4\pi}{3}$. Choice C is not the correct answer because it is not the correct reduction of the fraction. Choice D is not the correct answer because it is not the correct reduction of the fraction.

22. D: When you simplify $(\frac{\pi}{5}) \times (\frac{\pi}{180})$, you get $36°$. Choice A is not the correct answer because $10°$ is $\frac{\pi}{18}$. Choice B is not the correct answer because $20°$ is $\frac{\pi}{9}$. Choice C is not the correct answer because $30°$ is $\frac{\pi}{6}$.

23. C: When you simplify $(\frac{\pi}{6}) \times (\frac{\pi}{180})$, you get $30°$. Choice A is not the correct answer because $10°$ is $\frac{\pi}{18}$. Choice B is not the correct answer because $20°$ is $\frac{\pi}{9}$. Choice D is not the correct answer because $36°$ is $\frac{\pi}{5}$.

24. B: This answer is correct because $\frac{\pi}{9}$ reduces to $20°$. Choice A is not the correct answer because $10°$ is $\frac{\pi}{18}$. Choice C is not the correct answer because $25°$ is $\frac{5\pi}{36}$. Choice D is not the correct answer because $30°$ is $\frac{\pi}{6}$.

25. A: This answer is correct because $10°$ is $\frac{\pi}{18}$, when you multiply $10 \times (\frac{\pi}{180})$. Choice B is not the correct answer because $20°$ is $\frac{\pi}{9}$. Choice C is not the correct answer because $30°$ is $\frac{\pi}{6}$. Choice D is not the correct answer because $36°$ is $\frac{\pi}{5}$.

26. C: The formula for the length of an arc is $(central\ angle) \times (2\pi r) = (arc\ length) \times (360°)$, and $(36°)(2\pi 10) = (arc\ length) \times (360°)$, which reduces to 2π centimeters. Choice A is not the answer because the 2 is in the denominator. Choice B is not the answer since it was not multiplied by 2. Choice D is not the answer because it is double the correct arc length.

27. B: The formula for the length of an arc is $(central\ angle) \times (2\pi r) = (arc\ length) \times (360°)$, and $(72°)(2\pi 20) = (arc\ length) \times (360°)$, which reduces to 4π inches. Choice A is not the answer because it is double the correct arc length. Choice C is not correct since it is half of the correct arc length. Choice D is not the correct answer because it shows that the canceling of the numbers is not correct.

28. B: The formula for the length of an arc is $(central\ angle) \times (2\pi r) = (arc\ length) \times (360°)$ and $(20°)(2\pi 108) = (arc\ length) \times (360°)$. Choices A, C, and D, are not correct because they signify that the simplification was performed incorrectly.

29. D: The formula for the area of the circle is πr^2 and 5^2 is 25. Choice A is not the correct answer because that would be 2 times the radius. Choice B is not the correct answer because that would be 5×3. Choice C is not the correct answer because that would be 2^2 times the radius.

30. C: The formula for the area of the circle is πr^2 and 10^2 is 100. Choice A is not the correct answer because 10 is not squared. Choice B is not the correct answer because that is 2×10. Choice D is not the correct answer because that is $r^2 \times 2$.

31. A: The formula for the area of the circle is πr^2 and 9 squared is 81. Choice B is not the correct answer because that is 2×9. Choice C is not the correct answer because that is 9×10. Choice D is not the correct answer because that is simply the value of the radius.

32. B: The formula for the area of the circle is πr^2 and 13 squared is 169. Choice A is not the correct answer because that is 13×2. Choice C is not the correct answer because that is 13×10. Choice D is not the correct answer because that is $2 \times 13 \times 10$.

33. B: $Chord\ Length = radius \times \sin\frac{angle}{2}$, and $20 \times \sin$ of 60 is 10. Choice A is not the correct answer because it is the chord length formula divided by 4. Choice C is not the correct answer because it is the chord length plus 5. Choice D is not the correct answer because it is the chord length formula that has not been divided by 2.

34. C: $Chord\ Length = radius \times \sin\frac{angle}{2}$, and $30 \times \sin$ of 60 is 15. Choice A is not the correct answer because that is the radius divided by 6. Choice B is not the correct answer because that is the radius divided by 3. Choice D is not the correct answer because that is the radius minus 10.

35. D: The method to equate the two chord lengths is $3 + x + 2 = x + 3x + 2$, add like terms, $5 + x = 4x + 2$, solve for x ($x = 1$), and substitute 1 back into the equation. Choice A is not the correct answer because 1 is the solution for x, not the length of the chord. Choice B is not the correct answer because 2 is one of the terms of the chord length when adding like terms. Choice C is not the correct answer because 3 is only the coefficient of one of the terms when solving.

36. A: The method is to equate the two chord lengths: $4 + 2x + 2 = x + 3x + 2$, add the like terms, $6 + 2x = 4x + 2$, solve for $x(x = 2)$, and substitute 2 back into the equation. Choice B is not the correct answer because 2 is the solution for x, not the length of the chord. Choice C is not the correct answer because there is no 1 in the problem. Choice D is not the correct answer because 3 is only a coefficient in solving the equation.

Science

1. C: Molecules that are soluble in lipids, like fats, sterols, and vitamins (A, D, E and K), for example, are able to move in and out of a cell using passive transport. Water and oxygen are also able to move in and out of the cell without the use of cellular energy. Complex sugars and non-lipid soluble molecules are too large to move through the cell membrane without relying on active transport mechanisms. Molecules naturally move from areas of high concentration to those of lower concentration. It requires active transport to move molecules in the opposite direction, as suggested by Choice D.

2. A: Both types of cells are enclosed by plasma membranes with cytosol on the inside. Prokaryotes contain a nucleoid and do not have organelles; eukaryotes contain a nucleus enclosed by a membrane, as well as organelles.

3. B: During telophase, two nuclei form at each end of the cell and nuclear envelopes begin to form around each nucleus. The nucleoli reappear, and the chromosomes become less compact. The microtubules are broken down by the cell, and mitosis is complete. The process begins with prophase as the mitotic spindles begin to form from centrosomes. Prometaphase follows, with the breakdown of the nuclear envelope and the further condensing of the chromosomes. Next, metaphase occurs when the microtubules are stretched across the cell and the chromosomes align at the metaphase plate. Finally, in the last step before telophase, anaphase occurs as the sister chromatids break apart and form chromosomes.

4. D: Meiosis has the same phases as mitosis, except that they occur twice—once in meiosis I and once in meiosis II. During meiosis I, the cell splits into two. Each cell contains two sets of chromosomes. Next, during meiosis II, the two intermediate daughter cells divide again, producing four total haploid cells that each contain one set of chromosomes.

5. D: The naming of compounds focuses on the second element in a chemical compound. Elements from the non-metal category are written with an "ide" at the end. The compound CO has one carbon and one oxygen, so it is called carbon monoxide. Choice B represents that there are two oxygen atoms, and Choices A and B incorrectly alter the name of the first element, which should remain as carbon.

6. B: To solve this, the number of moles of NaCl needs to be calculated:

First, to find the mass of NaCl, the mass of each of the molecule's atoms is added together as follows:

$$23.0g \text{ (Na)} + 35.5g \text{ (Cl)} = 58.8g \text{ NaCl}$$

Next, the given mass of the substance is multiplied by one mole per total mass of the substance:

$$4.0g \text{ NaCl} \times (1 \text{ mol NaCl}/58.5g \text{ NaCl}) = 0.068 \text{ mol NaCl}$$

Finally, the moles are divided by the number of liters of the solution to find the molarity:

$$(0.068 \text{ mol NaCl})/(0.120L) = 0.57 \text{ M NaCl}$$

Choice A incorporates a miscalculation for the molar mass of NaCl, and Choices C and D both incorporate a miscalculation by not converting mL into liters (L), so they are incorrect by a factor of 10.

7. C: According to the *ideal gas law* ($PV = nRT$), if volume is constant, the temperature is directly related to the pressure in a system. Therefore, if the pressure increases, the temperature will increase in direct proportion. Choice A would not be possible, since the system is closed and a change is occurring, so the temperature will change. Choice B incorrectly exhibits an inverse relationship between pressure and temperature, or $P = 1/T$. Choice D is incorrect because even without actual values for the variables, the relationship and proportions can be determined.

8. A: According to Ohm's Law: $V = IR$, so using the given variables: $3.0 \text{ V} = I \times 6.0 \text{ } \Omega$

Solving for I: $I = 3.0 \text{ V}/6.0 \text{ } \Omega = 0.5 \text{ A}$

Choice B incorporates a miscalculation in the equation by multiplying 3.0 V by 6.0 Ω, rather than dividing these values. Choices C and D are labeled with the wrong units; Joules measure energy, not current.

9. A: The decimal point for this value is located after the final zero. Because the decimal is moved 12 places to the left in order to get it between the 8 and the 6, then the resulting exponent is positive, so Choice A is the correct answer. Choice B is false because the decimal has been moved in the wrong direction. Choice C is incorrect because the decimal has been moved an incorrect number of times. Choice D is false because this value is written to three significant figures, not two.

8,600,000,000,000
12 11 10 9 8 7 6 5 4 3 2 1

10. D: Leading zeros (those present after a decimal) are never significant, while all non-zero digits are significant. Therefore, in the value 0.00067, the only significant figures are 6 and 7, so this value has only two significant figures, making Choice D correct. Choices A, B, and C assume that all or some of the zeros are significant, so these options are incorrect.

11. B: The set of results is close to the actual value of the acceleration due to gravity, making the results accurate. However, there is a different value recorded every time, so the results aren't precise, which makes Choice B the correct answer.

12. A: To find the mean, the sum of the values can be calculated and then divided by the number of values. To report the result to the appropriate number of significant figures, the number of significant figures in which the values were given must be identified. In this case, every value is given at two significant figures. When the values are added and divided by four, they yield a value of 6.425. However, because the values are given in two significant figures, then the answer is 6.4. Choices B, C, and D give an incorrect number of significant figures.

$$\frac{3.2 + 7.5 + 9.6 + 5.4}{4} = 6.4$$

13. C: The graph shows that as the value of x increases, the value of y decreases, which is the definition of a negative correlation, so Choice C is correct. A positive correlation is when the value of y increases as the value of x increases, so Choice A is incorrect. Choices B and D both show no determinable relationship between two variables.

14. B: It's actually highly recommended to use substitutions for any harmful chemicals for educational purposes, so Choice B is the correct answer. Choices A, C, and D are all proper ways to handle chemicals and specimens.

15. A: Acids and bases should not be stored in metal, as they will corrode it. All the other listed substances can be stored in metal (note that dihydrogen monoxide is the scientific name for water).

16. D: Water's unique properties are due to intermolecular hydrogen bonding. These forces make water molecules "stick" to one another, which explains why water has unusually high cohesion and adhesion (sticking to each other and sticking to other surfaces). Cohesion can be seen in beads of dew. Adhesion can be seen when water sticks to the sides of a graduated cylinder to form a meniscus. The stickiness to neighboring molecules also increases surface tension, providing a very thin film that light things cannot penetrate, which is observed when leaves float in swimming pools. Water has a low freezing point, not a high freezing point, due to the fact that molecules have to have a very low kinetic energy to arrange themselves in the lattice-like structure found in ice, its solid form.

17. A: Catabolic reactions release energy and are exothermic. Catabolism breaks down complex molecules into simpler molecules. Anabolic reactions are just the opposite—they absorb energy in order to form complex molecules from simpler ones. Proteins, carbohydrates (polysaccharides), lipids, and nucleic acids are complex organic molecules synthesized by anabolic metabolism. The monomers of these organic compounds are amino acids, monosaccharides, triglycerides, and nucleotides.

18. C: Metabolic reactions utilize enzymes to decrease their activation energy. Enzymes that drive these reactions are protein catalysts. Their mechanism is sometimes referred to as the "lock-and-key" model. "Lock and key" references the fact that enzymes have exact specificity with their substrate (reactant) like a lock does to a key. The substrate binds to the enzyme snugly, the enzyme facilitates the reaction, and then product is formed while the enzyme is unchanged and ready to be reused.

19. B: The structure exclusively found in eukaryotic cells is the nucleus. Animal, plant, fungi, and protist cells are all eukaryotic. DNA is contained within the nucleus of eukaryotic cells, and they also have membrane-bound organelles that perform complex intracellular metabolic activities. Prokaryotic cells (archae and bacteria) do not have a nucleus or other membrane-bound organelles and are less complex than eukaryotic cells.

20. A: The Golgi complex, also known as the Golgi apparatus, is not found in the nucleus. Chromosomes, the nucleolus, and chromatin are all found within the nucleus of the cell. The Golgi apparatus is found in the cytoplasm and is responsible for protein maturation, the process of proteins folding into their secondary, tertiary, and quaternary configurations. The structure appears folded in membranous layers and is easily visible with microscopy. The Golgi apparatus packages proteins in vesicles for export out of the cell or to their cellular destination.

21. B: The mitochondria are cellular energy generators and the "powerhouses" of the cell. They provide cellular energy in the form of adenosine triphosphate (ATP). This process, called aerobic respiration, uses oxygen plus sugars, proteins, and fats to produce ATP, carbon dioxide, and water. Mitochondria contain their own DNA and ribosomes, which is significant because according to endosymbiotic theory, these structures provide evidence that they used to be independently-functioning prokaryotes.

22. B: Plastids are the photosynthesizing organelles of plants that are not found in animal cells. Plants have the ability to generate their own sugars through photosynthesis, a process where they use pigments to capture the sun's light energy. Chloroplasts are the most prevalent plastid, and chlorophyll is the light-absorbing pigment that absorbs all energy carried in photons except that of green light. This explains why the photosynthesizing parts of plants, predominantly leaves, appear green.

23. B: Diffusion and osmosis are examples of passive transport. Unlike active transport, passive transport does not require cellular energy. Diffusion is the movement of particles, such as ions, nutrients, or waste, from high concentration to low. Osmosis is the spontaneous movement of water from an area of high concentration to one of low concentration. Facilitated diffusion is another type of passive transport where particles move from high concentration to low concentration via a protein channel.

24. B: Phenotypes are observable traits, such as eye color, hair color, blood type, etc. They can also be biochemical or have physiological or behavioral traits. A genotype is the collective gene representation of an individual, whether the genes are expressed or not. Alleles are different forms of the same gene that code for specific traits, like blue eyes or brown eyes. In simple genetics, there are two forms of a gene: dominant and recessive. More complex genetics involves co-dominant, multiple alleles and sex-linked genes. The other answer choices are incorrect because gender is determined by the presence of an entire chromosome, the Y chromosome, and a karyotype is an image of all of an individual's chromosomes.

25. D: Reproductive cells are referred to as gametes: egg (female) and sperm (male). These cells have only 1 set of 23 chromosomes and are haploid so that when they combine during fertilization, the zygote has the correct diploid number, 46. Reproductive cell division is called meiosis, which is different from mitosis, the type of division process for body (somatic) cells.

26. A: The process of cell division in somatic is mitosis. In interphase, which precedes mitosis, cells prepare for division by copying their DNA. Once mitotic machinery has been assembled in interphase, mitosis occurs, which has four distinct phases: prophase, metaphase, anaphase, and telophase, followed by cytokinesis, which is the final splitting of the cytoplasm. The two diploid daughter cells are genetically identical to the parent cell.

27. D: Human gametes each contain 23 chromosomes. This is referred to as haploid—half the number of the original germ cell (46). Germ cells are diploid precursors of the haploid egg and sperm. Meiosis has two major phases, each of which is characterized by sub-phases similar to mitosis. In Meiosis I, the DNA of the parent cell is duplicated in interphase, just like in mitosis. Starting with prophase I, things become a little different. Two homologous chromosomes form a tetrad, cross over, and exchange genetic content. Each shuffled chromosome of the tetrad migrates to the cell's poles, and two haploid daughter cells are formed. In Meiosis II, each daughter undergoes another division more similar to mitosis (with the exception of the fact that there is no interphase), resulting in four genetically-different cells, each with only $\frac{1}{2}$ of the chromosomal material of the original germ cell.

28. A: The crossing over, or rearrangement of chromosomal sections in tetrads during meiosis, results in each gamete having a different combination of alleles than other gametes. *B* is incorrect because the presence of a Y chromosome determines gender. *C* is incorrect because it is improper separation in anaphase, not recombination, that causes non-disjunction. *D* is incorrect because transcription is an entirely different process involved in protein expression.

29. A: An alteration in the normal gene sequence is called a DNA point mutation. Mutations can be harmful, neutral, or even beneficial. Sometimes, as seen in natural selection, a genetic mutation can improve fitness, providing an adaptation that will aid in survival. DNA mutations can happen as a result of environmental damage, for example, from radiation or chemicals. Mutations can also happen during cell replication, as a result of incorrect pairing of complementary nucleotides by DNA polymerase. There are also chromosomal mutations as well, where entire segments of chromosomes can be deleted, inverted, duplicated, or sent or received from a different chromosome.

30. B: 50%. According to the Punnett square, the child has a 2 out of 4 chance of having A-type blood, since the dominant allele I^A is present in two of the four possible offspring. The O-type blood allele is masked by the A-type blood allele since it is recessive.

IA i	ii
IA i	ii

31. D: The building blocks of DNA are nucleotides. A nucleotide is a five-carbon sugar with a phosphate group and a nitrogenous base (Adenine, Guanine, Cytosine, and Thymine). DNA is a double helix and looks like a spiral ladder. Each side has a sugar/phosphate backbone, and the rungs of the ladder that connect the sides are the nitrogen bases. Adenine always pairs with thymine via two hydrogen bonds, and cytosine always pairs with guanine via three hydrogen bonds. The weak hydrogen bonds are important because they allow DNA to easily be opened for replication and transcription.

32. D: There are actually many different types of RNA. The three involved in protein synthesis are messenger RNA (mRNA), ribosomal RNA (rRNA), and transfer RNA (tRNA). Others, including small interfering RNA, micro RNA, and piwi associated RNA, are being investigated. Their known functions include gene regulation, facilitating chromosome wrapping, and unwrapping. RNA, unlike DNA, can be single stranded (mRNA, specifically), has a ribose sugar (rather than deoxyribose, like in DNA), and contains uracil (in place of thymine in DNA).

33. D: Equal sharing of electrons is correct. In water, the electronegative oxygen sucks in the electrons of the two hydrogen atoms, making the oxygen slightly negatively-charged and the hydrogen atoms slightly positively-charged. This unequal sharing is called "polarity." This polarity is responsible for the slightly-positive hydrogen atoms from one molecule being attracted to a slightly-negative oxygen in a different molecule, creating a weak intermolecular force called a hydrogen bond, so *A* and *B* are true. *C* is also true, because this unique hydrogen bonding creates intermolecular forces that literally hold molecules with low enough kinetic energy (at low temperatures) to be held apart at "arm's length" (really, the length of the hydrogen bonds). This makes ice less dense than liquid, which explains why ice floats, a very unique property of water. *D* is the only statement that is false, so it is the correct answer.

34. D: Cellular respiration is the term used for the set of metabolic reactions that convert chemical bonds to energy in the form of ATP. All respiration starts with glycolysis in the cytoplasm, and in the presence of oxygen, the process will continue to the mitochondria. In a series of oxidation/reduction reactions, primarily glucose will be broken down so that the energy contained within its bonds can be transferred to the smaller ATP molecules. It's like having a $100 bill (glucose) as opposed to having one hundred $1 bills. This is beneficial to the organism because it allows energy to be distributed throughout the cell very easily in smaller packets of energy.

When glucose is broken down, its electrons and hydrogen atoms are involved in oxidative phosphorylation in order to make ATP, while its carbon and oxygen atoms are released as carbon dioxide. Anaerobic respiration does not occur frequently in humans, but during rigorous exercise, lack of available oxygen in the muscles can lead to anaerobic ATP production in a process called lactic acid fermentation. Alcohol fermentation is another type of anaerobic respiration that occurs in yeast. Anaerobic respiration is extremely less efficient than aerobic respiration, as it has a net yield of 2ATP, while aerobic respiration's net yield exceeds 30 ATP.

35. D: All statements are true, but nothing can happen without the message being available; thus, Choice *D* must occur first. After the copy is made in transcription (*D*), Choice *B* occurs because mRNA has to be processed before being exported into the cytoplasm. Once it has reached the cytoplasm, Choice *A* occurs as mRNA is pulled into the ribosome. Finally, Choice *C* occurs, and tRNA delivers amino acids one at a time until the full polypeptide has been created. At that point, the baby protein (polypeptide) will be processed and folded in the ER and Golgi.

36. B: Punctuated equilibrium is the concept that evolution is comprised of eras of no change, (called "stasis") peppered with short period of rapid change, often resulting in speciation. The theory was researched and proposed by Stephen J. Gould and Niles Eldridge in opposition to Darwin's idea of gradualism. Gradualism maintains that evolution progresses at a steady, gradual pace without sudden new developments.

37. A: All the other answer choices are functions of lipids. Choice *B* is true because steroid hormones are lipid based. Long-term energy is one of the most important functions of lipids, so *C* is true. *D* is also true because the cell membrane is not only composed of a lipid bilayer, but it also has cholesterol (another lipid) embedded within it to regulate membrane fluidity.

38. D: Ribosomes are the structures responsible for protein synthesis using amino acids delivered by tRNA molecules. They are numerous within the cell and can take up as much as 25% of the cell. Ribosomes are found free-floating in the cytoplasm and also attached to the rough endoplasmic reticulum, which resides alongside the nucleus. Ribosomes translate messenger RNA into chains of amino acids that become proteins. Ribosomes themselves are made of protein as well as rRNA. Choice *B* might be an attractive choice, since the Golgi is the site of protein maturation; however, it is not where proteins are synthesized. Choice *A* might be an attractive choice as well because DNA provides the instructions for proteins to be made, but DNA does not make the protein itself.

39. D: DNA and RNA each contain four nitrogenous bases, three of which they have in common: adenine, guanine, and cytosine. Thymine is only found in DNA, and uracil is only found in RNA. Adenine interacts with uracil in RNA, and with thymine in DNA. Guanine always pairs with cytosine in both DNA and RNA.

40. B: Dominant alleles are considered to have stronger phenotypes and, when mixed with recessive alleles, will mask the recessive trait. The recessive trait would only appear as the phenotype when the allele combination is "aa" because a dominant allele is not present to mask it.

41. A: Speciation is the method by which one species splits into two or more species. In allopatric speciation, one population is divided into two subpopulations. If a drought occurs and a large lake becomes divided into two smaller lakes, each lake is left with its own population that cannot intermingle with the population of the other lake. When the genes of these two subpopulations are no longer mixing with each other, new mutations can arise and natural selection can take place.

42. C: In the Linnean system, organisms are classified as follows, moving from comprehensive and specific similarities to fewer and more general similarities: species, genus, family, order, class, phylum, kingdom, and domain. A popular mnemonic device to remember the Linnean system is "Dear King Philip came over for good soup."

43. A: Fungal cells have a cell wall, similar to plant cells; however, they use oxygen as a source of energy and cannot perform photosynthesis. Because they do not perform photosynthesis, fungal cells do not contain chloroplasts.

44. A: Roots are responsible for absorbing water and nutrients that will get transported up through the plant. They also anchor the plant to the ground. Photosynthesis occurs in leaves, stems transport materials through the plant and support the plant body, and phloem moves sugars downward to the leaves.

45. D: Tropism is a response to stimuli that causes the plant to grow toward or away from the stimuli. Hydrotropism is a response to a change in water concentration. Phototropism is a reaction to light that causes plants to grow toward the source of the light. Thermotropism is a response to changes in temperature. Gravitropism is a response to gravity that causes roots to follow the pull of gravity and grow downward, but also causes plant shoots to act against gravity and grow upward.

46. B: The respiratory system mediates the exchange of gas between the air and the circulating blood, mainly by the act of breathing. It filters, warms, and humidifies the air that gets breathed in and then passes it into the blood stream. The digestive system transforms food and liquids into energy and helps excrete waste from the body. Eliminating waste via the kidneys and bladder is a function of the urinary system.

47. D: Arteries carry oxygen-rich blood from the heart to the other tissues of the body. Veins carry oxygen-poor blood back to the heart. Intestines carry digested food through the body. Bronchioles are passageways that carry air from the nose and mouth to the lungs.

48. A: The skeletal system consists of the 206 bones that make up the skeleton, as well as the cartilage, ligaments, and other connective tissues that stabilize the bones. The skeletal system provides structural support for the entire body, a framework for the soft tissues and organs to attach to, and acts as a protective barrier for some organs, such as the ribs protecting the heart and lungs, and the vertebrae protecting the spinal cord. The muscular system includes skeletal muscles, cardiac muscle, and the smooth muscles found on the inside of blood vessels. The endocrine system uses ductless glands to produce hormones that help maintain hemostasis, and the reproductive system is responsible for the production of egg and sperm cells.

49. C: Population dynamics looks at the composition of populations, including size and age, and the biological and environmental processes that cause changes. These can include immigration, emigration, births, and deaths.

50. A: Ecosystems are maintained by cycling the energy and nutrients that they obtain from external sources. The process can be diagramed in a food web, which represents the feeding relationship between the species in a community. A phylogenetic tree shows inferred evolutionary relationships among species and is similar to the fossil record. A pedigree chart shows occurrences of phenotypes of a particular gene through the generations of an organism.

51. D: The weight of an object is equal to the mass of the object multiplied by gravity. According to Newton's Second Law of Motion, $F = m \times a$. Weight is the force resulting from a given situation, so the mass of the object needs to be multiplied by the acceleration of gravity on Earth: $W = m \times g$. Choice A is incorrect because, according to Newton's first law, all objects exert some force on each other, based on their distance from each other and their masses. This is seen in planets, which affect each other's paths and those of their moons. Choice B is incorrect because an object in motion or at rest can have inertia; inertia is the resistance of a physical object to change its state of motion. Choice C is incorrect because the mass of an object is a measurement of how much substance there is to the object, while the weight is gravity's effect of the mass.

52. B: A decomposition reaction breaks down a compound into its constituent elemental components. Choice A is incorrect because a synthesis reaction joins two or more elements into a single compound. Choice C, an organic reaction, is not possible, since it needs carbon and hydrogen for a reaction. Choice D, oxidation/reduction (redox or half) reaction, is incorrect because it involves the loss of electrons from one species (oxidation) and the gain of electrons to the other species (reduction). There is no notation of this occurring within the given reaction, so it is incorrect.

53. C:

$$2Na + Cl_2 \longrightarrow 2NaCl$$

The number of each element must be equal on both sides of the equation:

Choice C is the only correct option: $2Na + Cl_2 \rightarrow 2NaCl$

2 Na + 2 Cl does equal 2 Na + 2 Cl (the number of sodium atoms and chlorine atoms match)

Choice A: $Na + Cl_2 \rightarrow NaCl$

1 Na + 2 Cl does not equal 1 Na + 1 Cl (the number of chlorine atoms do not match)

Choice B: $2Na + Cl_2 \rightarrow NaCl$

2 Na + 2 Cl does not equal 1 Na + 1 Cl (neither the number of sodium atoms nor chlorine atoms match)

Choice *D*: 2Na + 2Cl$_2$ → 2NaCl

2 Na + 4 Cl does not equal 2 Na + 2 Cl (the number of chlorine atoms do not match)

English & Language Usage

1. B: Parentheses indicate that the information contained within carries less weight or importance than the surrounding text. The word *essential* makes Choice *A* false. The information, though relevant, is not essential, and the paragraph could survive without it. For Choice *C*, the information is not repeated at any point, and, therefore, is not redundant. For Choice *D*, the information is placed next to his height, which is relevant. Placing it anywhere else would make it out of place.

2. A: *Principals* are the leaders of a school. *Principles* indicate values, morals, or ideology. For Choice *B*, the words are reversed. For Choices *C* and *D*, both answers are misspelled, regardless of position.

3. C: *His* or *her* is correct. *Each* indicates the need for a singular pronoun, and because the charts belong to the patients, they must be possessive as well. To indicate that the group of patients could include males and females, *his* and *her* must be included. For Choice *A*, *there* is plural. For Choice *B*, *there* is an adverb, not a pronoun. For Choice *D*, *the people's* is collective plural, not singular.

4. B: *Imminent* means impending or happening soon. The man fears going to the zoo because a bomb might soon be detonated. For Choice *A*, *eminent* means of a high rank or status. For Choice *C*, *emanate* means to originate from. For Choice *D*, *amanita* is a type of fungus.

5. C: Semicolons can function as conjunctions. When used thus, they take the place of *and*, joining two independent clauses together. Choice *A* is incorrect because colons introduce lists or a final, emphasized idea. The independent clauses in this example carry equal emphasis. Choice *B* is an example of a run-on sentence. Commas may not be used to join two independent clauses. Choice *D* is also a run-on sentence. There's not punctuation of any type to indicate two separate clauses that can stand on their own.

6. C: This answer includes two independent clauses that could stand on their own. To test this, try separating each sentence and putting a period at the end. For Choice *C*, since each clause includes its own noun and verb, they each could stand independently of one another. For Choice *A*, there are two nouns, Tod and Elissa, and three verbs: went, got, and slept. This sentence cannot be separated into independent clauses. Choice *B* begins with a subordinate conjunction, making one sentence rely on the other. The same goes for Choice *D*; *while Marge slept* is a dependent clause.

7. C: *Ran* functions as a verb and is conjugated with the noun *lecture*. For Choice *A*, *engaging* acts as a gerund and an adjective, describing what type of lecture. For Choice *B*, *though* can act as a conjunction or adverb, but not a verb. For Choice *D*, *over* is an adverb that describes *ran*.

8. B: Adverbs describe verbs or adjectives. In this instance, *almost* describes *arrived*, the verb. Adverbs answer questions like *how* or *where* and here *almost* describes *how* he arrived. For *A*, *arrived* is a past-tense verb. For *C*, *irritated* functions as an adjective, describing Dave's boss. *Rest* (Choice *D*) is a noun, evidenced by the article, *the*, before it.

9. D: Summer is generic, so it doesn't require capitalization. Titles (*President*) are capitalized when they're specific and precede the person's name. It's similar to saying *Mr.* or *Mrs.*, followed by a person's name. Choice *A* is incorrect because *advanced history* should not be capitalized. It's already been established that *History 220* is the official name of the class, and *advanced* is indicating that the class is rigorous, especially in contrast to *entry-level*. Choice *B* is incorrect because *professor* should not be capitalized. It follows the name of the individual, and, therefore, does not qualify as a title. Choice *C* is incorrect because *army* and *navy* are specific to the British Empire, and, therefore, function as proper nouns.

10. D: This passage displays clarity (the author states precisely what he or she intended), fluency (the sentences run smoothly together), and parallelism (words are used in a similar fashion to help provide rhythm). Choice *A* lacks parallelism. When the author states, "the hero acts without thinking, is living in the moment, and is repressing physical and emotional pain," the words *acts, is living* and *is repressing* are in different tenses, and, consequently, jarring to one's ears. Choice *B* runs on endlessly in the first half ("Ernest Hemingway is probably the most noteworthy of expatriate authors since his concise writing style is void of emotion and stream of consciousness and has had a lasting impact on Americans which has resonated to this very day, and Hemingway's novels are much like in American cinema.") It demands some type of pause and strains the readers' eyes. The second half of the passage is choppy: "The hero acts. He doesn't think. He lives in the moment. He represses physical and emotional pain." For Choice *C*, leaving out *expatriate* is, first, vague, and second, alters the meaning. The correct version claims that Hemingway was the most notable of the expatriate authors while the second version claims he's the most notable of any author *ever*, a very bold claim indeed. Also, leaving out *stream of* in "stream of consciousness" no longer references the non-sequential manner in which most people think. Instead, this version sounds like all the characters in the novel are in a coma!

11. A: Books are italicized, like *Frankenstein*, and smaller works are put in quotation marks. A direct quotation takes a single set of quotation marks (" ") and a quote within a quote take a single set (' '). Choice *B* is incorrect because *Frankenstein* should be italicized, not put in quotation marks. In Choice *C*, the double and single-set quotation marks should be reversed. In Choice *D*, the comma is missing before the first quotation mark, and the period for the quote within a quote is on the outside of the quotation mark, not the inside. Punctuation belongs inside the quotation marks, regardless of whether it a single or double set.

12. B: Indefinite pronouns such as *everyone* always take the singular. The key is to delete unnecessary language mentally ("who has ever owned a pet and hasn't had help"), which allows one to better test the conjugation between noun and verb. In this case, *everyone* and *knows* are joined. Choice *A* is incorrect because *each* (another indefinite pronoun) is singular while the verb *have* is plural. In Choice *C*, *neither* is indefinite, so *is* should be *has*, not *have*. In Choice *D*, *One*, which is indefinite, is the noun. The prepositional phrase "of the very applauded and commended lecturers" can be removed from the sentence. Therefore, the singular *is* is needed, not *are*.

13. D: *Distraught* is an adjective because it describes *what* Sara (the noun) looks like. In Choice *A*, *never* is an adverb that modifies *is*. In Choice *B*, *after* is a preposition because it occurs before a noun, *class*, and establishes a relationship with the rest of the sentence. *Mess* (Choice *D*) is a noun.

14. C: Both second and third person points of view are represented. The phrases *one should have* and *it is* are in the third person. Typical third-person subjects include *he, she, him, her, they, one, person, people*, and *someone*. Second person voice is indicated in the second half of the passage by the words *you* and *your*. Second person is simple to identify because it is the *you* voice, in which the reader is directly addressed.

15. B: The word *conscience* means a sense of right and wrong. *Conscious* (Choice A) refers to a state of being awake and alert. *Consensus* (Choice C) means an opinion shared by many, and a *census* (Choice D) is a count of an area's population.

16. B: A simple sentence must contain three things: the subject, the verb, and the completed idea or thought. Once the nonessential clause "who is not yet sixty" is removed, one is left with, "Ted still easily fishes and camps, too." The combination of the verbs *fishes* and *camps* are known as compound verbs, but because there are no independent or dependent clauses combined, it is still considered simple. For Choice A, there's an independent clause ("Ted loves to rock climb") and a dependent clause ("even though he tore his rotator cuff.") *Even though* functions as a subordinate conjunction. For Choice C, there's two independent clauses ("Ted loves the outdoors" and "his wife is a homebody") joined by the compound conjunction *but*. For Choice D, there's two independent clauses ("Ted will also be retired soon" and "he likes to stay busy") joined with the conjunctive adverb *nevertheless*.

17. D: Here, the rules of plural possessive are followed, placing the apostrophe outside the *s*. The outside apostrophe confirms that there are multiple *businesses*, not just one, entertaining many *clients*. In Choice A, the word *women* is plural, so the apostrophe belongs before the added *s*; the correct usage is *women's*. For Choice B, knowing how to use *it's* versus *its* is critical. *It's* is always a contraction while *its* always shows ownership. In Choice C, the possessive is not in use at all.

18. C: For the prefix *anti-* to work in both situations, it must have the same meaning, one that generalizes to any word in the English language. *Oppose* makes sense in both instances. Antibiotics *oppose* bacteria, and antisocials *oppose* society. Choice A is illogical. *Reducing* the number of bacteria is somewhat logical, but *reducing* society doesn't make sense when considering the definition of antisocial. Choice B is not the best match for bacteria. *Revolt*, a word normally reserved for human opposition, sounds odd when paired with bacteria. Choice D might work for antibiotic (without bacteria) but doesn't work for antisocial (without society).

19. D: Shape is the best answer. If *conform* means to adjust behavior, *shape* could replace *conform*, as in the behavior was *re-shaped* or modified. The same goes for *inform*. New information *re-shapes* how one thinks about the world. Also, the word *shape* gives rise to the abstract idea that both behavior and information are malleable, like modeling clay, and can be molded into new forms. Choice A (*match*) works for *conform* (matching to society), but it doesn't work for *inform* (one cannot *match* information to a person). Choice B (*relay*) doesn't work for *conform* (there's no way to pass on new behavior), but it does work for *inform*, as to pass on new information. Choice C (*negate*) works for neither *conform* (the behavior is not being completely cancelled out) nor *inform* (the information is not being rescinded).

20. B: To arrive at the best answer (*surly*), all the character traits for Cindy must be analyzed. She's described as *happy* ("always has a smile on her face"), *kind* ("volunteers at the local shelter"), and *patient* ("no one has ever seen her angry"). Since Cindy's husband is the *opposite* of her, these adjectives must be converted to antonyms. Someone who is *surly* is *unhappy*, *rude*, and *impatient*. Choice A (*stingy*) is too narrow of a word. Someone could be *happy* and *kind*, for instance, but still be *stingy*. For Choice C, *scared*, to be plausible, the rest of the passage would need instances of Cindy being *bold* or *courageous*. Though she's certainly *kind* and *helpful*, none of those traits are modeled. Choice D (*shy*) also doesn't match. Someone who is *shy* could still be *happy*, *kind*, and *patient*.

21: A: *Grasp* is the best answer. It's important both in the New World and in Africa to ambulate or *move* (the word is used more than once), but only in the New World must mammals deal with dense vegetation and foliage. Choice B (*punch*) is incorrect because punching is unrelated to dealing with dense vegetation. *Prehensile tails* are designed to *grasp*. It's established in *both* environments that *movement* is critical to survival. Choice *C* (*move*) applies, again, to both jungle and savannah environments. Choice *D* (*walk*) would be applicable to savannahs, not environments populated with dense vegetation.

22. A: First person is the point of view represented. First person is known as the "I" voice. There are no "I's" in this passage, but the words *we* and *our* indicate first person plural. *We*, rationally, includes *I* and *other people*. *Our*, plural possessive, includes *mine* and *other's*. There is no evidence of second person (*you* voice), or third person (he, she, they). The narrator here is the "I," which means they are writing in first person.

23. B: "Make sure to clock out after your shift is through," includes both an independent and dependent clause. "Make sure to clock out" is the independent clause while "after your shift is through" is the dependent clause. *After* is the subordinate conjunction in this instance. Choice *A* is incorrect because "To make your fruit last longer" is a prepositional phrase, not a clause. "Keep it out of the sunlight" is an independent clause as well as an imperative command. For Choice *C*, "making a good fire" is considered a gerund phrase and is followed by the compound verbs *using* and *stacking*. Since there are no compound or complex sentences joined, it's considered a simple sentence. "Whenever possible," is an adverbial clause, not a dependent clause, so it's not classified as a complex sentence when paired with an independent clause ("Make sure to yield to oncoming traffic"). It, too, is a simple sentence.

24. B: *Accent* refers to the regional manner or style in which one speaks. *Ascent* refers to the act of rising or climbing. *Assent* means consensus or agreement. The people of Scotland have unique *accents* or dialects, and they're used to lofty *ascents* or climbs.

25. B: In Choice *B*, the word *Uncle* should not be capitalized, because it is not functioning as a proper noun. If the word named a specific uncle, such as *Uncle Jerry*, then it would be considered a proper noun and should be capitalized. Choice *A* correctly capitalizes the proper noun *East Coast*, and does not capitalize *winter*, which functions as a common noun in the sentence. Choice *C* correctly capitalizes the name of a specific college course, which is considered a proper noun. Choice *D* correctly capitalizes the proper noun *Jersey Shore*.

26. C: In Choice *C*, *avid* is functioning as an adjective that modifies the word photographer. *Avid* describes the photographer Julia Robinson's style. The words *time* and *photographer* are functioning as nouns, and the word *capture* is functioning as a verb in the sentence. Other words functioning as adjectives in the sentence include *local*, *business*, and *spare*, as they all describe the nouns they precede.

27. A: Choice *A* is correctly punctuated because it uses a semicolon to join two independent clauses that are related in meaning. Each of these clauses could function as an independent sentence. Choice *B* is incorrect because the conjunction is not preceded by a comma. A comma and conjunction should be used together to join independent clauses. Choice *C* is incorrect because a comma should only be used to join independent sentences when it also includes a coordinating conjunction such as *and* or *so*. Choice *D* does not use punctuation to join the independent clauses, so it is considered a fused (same as a run-on) sentence.

28. C: Choice *C* is a compound sentence because it joins two independent clauses with a comma and the coordinating conjunction *and*. The sentences in Choices *B* and *D* include one independent clause and one dependent clause, so they are complex sentences, not compound sentences. The sentence in

Choice *A* has both a compound subject, *Alex and Shane*, and a compound verb, *spent and took*, but the entire sentence itself is one independent clause.

ATI TEAS Practice Test #3

Reading

1. Xavier <u>propagated</u> his belief that dragons were real to his friends gathered around the campfire. Which of the following words could most logically replace the underlined word without altering the intent of the sentence?
   - a. Shouted
   - b. Expressed
   - c. Persuaded
   - d. Whispered

2. Which of the following statements least supports the argument that the American economy is healthy?
   - a. The United States' Gross Domestic Product (GDP), which is the measure of all the goods and services produced in a country, increased by two percent last year.
   - b. Unemployment is the lowest it's been in over a decade due to a spike in job creation.
   - c. Average household income just hit a historical high point for the twentieth consecutive quarter.
   - d. Last year, the output of the United States' manufacturing sector decreased despite repeated massive investments by both the private and public sectors.

The next three questions are based on the following table. The Dewey Decimal System is a library classification system.

The Dewey Decimal Classes
000 Computer science, information, and general works
100 Philosophy and psychology
200 Religion
300 Social sciences
400 Languages
500 Science and mathematics
600 Technical and applied science
700 Arts and recreation
800 Literature
900 History, geography, and biography

3. Teddy has been assigned to write a history paper about the United States during the Cold War. His teacher advised him to read some of the works of Noam Chomsky, an American linguist, philosopher, social scientist, cognitive scientist, historian, social critic, and political activist. Teddy was not sure where to begin, so he consulted the Dewey Decimal classes. While not all inclusive, what choice of three classes would likely be the most useful?
   - a. 100, 300, 700
   - b. 100, 300, 800
   - c. 100, 400, 900
   - d. 200, 300, 900

4. While researching Chomsky's many theories and arguments, Teddy became interested in post-World War II anarchism, a social science theory asserting the political philosophy that rejects a compulsory government. He wants to find the most appropriate works related to the subject. Which section of the library is the most likely to contain the relevant books?
    a. 000
    b. 200
    c. 300
    d. 900

5. Also during his research, Teddy discovered information about Chomsky's Jewish heritage, and he wants to research traditional Judaism as practiced in the early twentieth century. Which section of the library would most likely contain the most relevant information?
    a. 100
    b. 200
    c. 300
    d. 900

6. Which of the following statements best describes Samuel's sample size?
    a. The sample is biased because he has firsthand experience and personal knowledge of its participants.
    b. The sample contains too few members to make meaningful claims applicable to a large group.
    c. The sample contains too many members to understand the context and specifics of any given student's situation.
    d. The sample is unbiased and appropriately sized to draw conclusions on the role of parental supervision in education.

The next question is based on the following passage.

Annabelle Rice started having trouble sleeping. Her biological clock was suddenly amiss and she began to lead a nocturnal schedule. She thought her insomnia was due to spending nights writing a horror story, but then she realized that even the idea of going outside into the bright world scared her to bits. She concluded she was now suffering from heliophobia.

7. Which of the following most accurately describes the meaning of the underlined word in the sentence above?
    a. Fear of dreams
    b. Fear of sunlight
    c. Fear of strangers
    d. Anxiety spectrum disorder

The next question is based on the following directions.

Follow these instructions in chronological order to transform the word into something new.
    1. Start with the word LOATHING.
    2. Eliminate the first and last letter in the starting word.
    3. Eliminate all the vowels, except I, from the word.
    4. Eliminate the letter H from the word.

8. What new word has been spelled?
   a. TON
   b. THIN
   c. TIN
   d. TAN

9. Which of these descriptions gives the most detailed and objective support for the claim that drinking and driving is unsafe?
   a. A dramatized television commercial reenacting a fatal drinking and driving accident, including heart-wrenching testimonials from loved ones
   b. The Department of Transportation's press release noting the additional drinking and driving special patrol units that will be on the road during the holiday season
   c. Congressional written testimony on the number of drinking and driving incidents across the country and their relationship to underage drinking statistics, according to experts
   d. A highway bulletin warning drivers of penalties associated with drinking and driving

The next question is based on the following passage.

A famous children's author recently published a historical fiction novel under a pseudonym; however, it did not sell as many copies as her children's books. In her earlier years, she had majored in history and earned a graduate degree in Antebellum American History, which is the time frame of her new novel. Critics praised this newest work far more than the children's series that made her famous. In fact, her new novel was nominated for the prestigious Albert J. Beveridge Award, but still isn't selling like her children's books, which fly off the shelves because of her name alone.

10. Which one of the following statements might be accurately inferred based on the above passage?
    a. The famous children's author produced an inferior book under her pseudonym.
    b. The famous children's author is the foremost expert on Antebellum America.
    c. The famous children's author did not receive the bump in publicity for her historical novel that it would have received if it were written under her given name.
    d. People generally prefer to read children's series than historical fiction.

The next four questions are based on the following passage.

Smoking is Terrible
Smoking tobacco products is terribly destructive. A single cigarette contains over 4,000 chemicals, including 43 known carcinogens and 400 deadly toxins. Some of the most dangerous ingredients include tar, carbon monoxide, formaldehyde, ammonia, arsenic, and DDT. Smoking can cause numerous types of cancer including throat, mouth, nasal cavity, esophagus, stomach, pancreas, kidney, bladder, and cervical.

Cigarettes contain a drug called nicotine, one of the most addictive substances known to man. Addiction is defined as a compulsion to seek the substance despite negative consequences. According to the National Institute of Drug Abuse, nearly 35 million smokers expressed a desire to quit smoking in 2015; however, more than 85 percent of those addicts will not achieve their goal. Almost all smokers regret picking up that first cigarette. You would be wise to learn from their mistake if you have not yet started smoking.

According to the U.S. Department of Health and Human Services, 16 million people in the United States presently suffer from a smoking-related condition and nearly nine million suffer from a serious smoking-related illness. According to the Centers for Disease Control and Prevention (CDC), tobacco products cause nearly six million deaths per year. This number is projected to rise to over eight million deaths by 2030. Smokers, on average, die ten years earlier than their nonsmoking peers.

In the United States, local, state, and federal governments typically tax tobacco products, which leads to high prices. Nicotine addicts sometimes pay more for a pack of cigarettes than for a few gallons of gas. Additionally, smokers tend to stink. The smell of smoke is all-consuming and creates a pervasive nastiness. Smokers also risk staining their teeth and fingers with yellow residue from the tar.

Smoking is deadly, expensive, and socially unappealing. Clearly, smoking is not worth the risks.

11. Which of the following best describes the passage?
    a. Narrative
    b. Persuasive
    c. Expository
    d. Technical

12. Which of the following statements most accurately summarizes the passage?
    a. Tobacco is less healthy than many alternatives.
    b. Tobacco is deadly, expensive, and socially unappealing, and smokers would be much better off kicking the addiction.
    c. In the United States, local, state, and federal governments typically tax tobacco products, which leads to high prices.
    d. Tobacco products shorten smokers' lives by ten years and kill more than six million people per year.

13. The author would be most likely to agree with which of the following statements?
    a. Smokers should only quit cold turkey and avoid all nicotine cessation devices.
    b. Other substances are more addictive than tobacco.
    c. Smokers should quit for whatever reason that gets them to stop smoking.
    d. People who want to continue smoking should advocate for a reduction in tobacco product taxes.

14. Which of the following represents an opinion statement on the part of the author?
    a. According to the Centers for Disease Control and Prevention (CDC), tobacco products cause nearly six million deaths per year.
    b. Nicotine addicts sometimes pay more for a pack of cigarettes than a few gallons of gas.
    c. They also risk staining their teeth and fingers with yellow residue from the tar.
    d. Additionally, smokers tend to stink. The smell of smoke is all-consuming and creates a pervasive nastiness.

The next question is based on the following passage.

In 2015, 28 countries, including Estonia, Portugal, Slovenia, and Latvia, scored significantly higher than the United States on standardized high school math tests. In the 1960s, the United States consistently ranked first in the world. Today, the United States spends more than $800 billion dollars on education, which exceeds the next highest country by more than $600 billion dollars. The United States also leads the world in spending per school-aged child by an enormous margin.

15. If these statements above are factual, which of the following statements must be correct?
    a. Outspending other countries on education has benefits beyond standardized math tests.
    b. The United States' education system is corrupt and broken.
    c. The standardized math tests are not representative of American academic prowess.
    d. Spending more money does not guarantee success on standardized math tests.

16. At the top of an encyclopedia's page are the following two guide terms: kingcraft and klieg light. Which one of the following words will be found on this page?
    a. Kleptomania
    b. Knead
    c. Kinesthesia
    d. Kickback

17. Which of the following is a primary source?
    a. A critic's summary and review of a new book on the life of Abraham Lincoln
    b. A peer-reviewed scientific journal's table of contents
    c. A report containing the data, summary, and conclusions of a recent gene splicing study
    d. A news article quoting recent groundbreaking research into curing cancer

The next question is based on the following passage.

Cynthia keeps to a strict vegetarian diet, which is part of her religion. She absolutely cannot have any meat or fish dishes. This is more than a preference; her body has never developed the enzymes to process meat or fish, so she becomes violently ill if she accidentally eats any of the offending foods.

Cynthia is attending a full day event at her college next week. When at an event that serves meals, she always likes to bring a platter of vegetarian food for herself and to share with other attendees who have similar dietary restrictions. She requested a menu in advance to determine when her platter might be most useful to vegetarians. Here is the menu:

Breakfast: Hazelnut coffee or English breakfast tea, French toast, eggs, and bacon strips
Lunch: Assorted sandwiches (vegetarian options available), French fries, and baked beans
Cocktail hour: Alcoholic beverages, fruit, and cheese
Dinner: Roasted pork loin, seared trout, and bacon-bit topped macaroni and cheese

18. If Cynthia wants to pick the meal where there would be the least options for her and fellow vegetarians, during what meal should she bring the platter?
    a. Breakfast
    b. Lunch
    c. Cocktail hour
    d. Dinner

The next three questions are based on the following passage.

George Washington emerged out of the American Revolution as an unlikely champion of liberty. On June 14, 1775, the Second Continental Congress created the Continental Army, and John Adams, serving in the Congress, nominated Washington to be its first commander. Washington fought under the British during the French and Indian War, and his experience and prestige proved instrumental to the American war effort. Washington provided invaluable leadership, training, and strategy during the Revolutionary War. He emerged from the war as the embodiment of liberty and freedom from tyranny.

After vanquishing the heavily favored British forces, Washington could have pronounced himself as the autocratic leader of the former colonies without any opposition, but he famously refused and returned to his Mount Vernon plantation. His restraint proved his commitment to the fledgling state's republicanism. Washington was later unanimously elected as the first American president. But it is Washington's farewell address that cemented his legacy as a visionary worthy of study.

In 1796, President Washington issued his farewell address by public letter. Washington enlisted his good friend, Alexander Hamilton, in drafting his most famous address. The letter expressed Washington's faith in the Constitution and rule of law. He encouraged his fellow Americans to put aside partisan differences and establish a national union. Washington warned Americans against meddling in foreign affairs and entering military alliances. Additionally, he stated his opposition to national political parties, which he considered partisan and counterproductive.

Americans would be wise to remember Washington's farewell, especially during presidential elections when politics hits a fever pitch. They might want to question the political institutions that were not planned by the Founding Fathers, such as the nomination process and political parties themselves.

19. Which of the following statements is logically based on the information contained in the passage above?
    a. George Washington's background as a wealthy landholder directly led to his faith in equality, liberty, and democracy.
    b. George Washington would have opposed America's involvement in the Second World War.
    c. George Washington would not have been able to write as great a farewell address without the assistance of Alexander Hamilton.
    d. George Washington would probably not approve of modern political parties.

20. Which of the following statements is the best description of the author's purpose in writing this passage about George Washington?
    a. To inform American voters about a Founding Father's sage advice on a contemporary issue and explain its applicability to modern times
    b. To introduce George Washington to readers as a historical figure worthy of study
    c. To note that George Washington was more than a famous military hero
    d. To convince readers that George Washington is a hero of republicanism and liberty

21. In which of the following materials would the author be the most likely to include this passage?
    a. A history textbook
    b. An obituary
    c. A fictional story
    d. A newspaper editorial

The next question is based on the following conversation between a scientist and a politician.

Scientist: Last year was the warmest ever recorded in the last 134 years. During that time period, the ten warmest years have all occurred since 2000. This correlates directly with the recent increases in carbon dioxide as large countries like China, India, and Brazil continue developing and industrializing. No longer do just a handful of countries burn massive amounts of carbon-based fossil fuels; it is quickly becoming the case throughout the whole world as technology and industry spread.

Politician: Yes, but there is no causal link between increases in carbon emissions and increasing temperatures. The link is tenuous and nothing close to certain. We need to wait for all of the data before drawing hasty conclusions. For all we know, the temperature increase could be entirely natural. I believe the temperatures also rose dramatically during the dinosaurs' time, and I do not think they were burning any fossil fuels back then.

22. What is one point on which the scientist and politician agree?
    a. Burning fossil fuels causes global temperatures to rise.
    b. Global temperatures are increasing.
    c. Countries must revisit their energy policies before it's too late.
    d. Earth's climate naturally goes through warming and cooling periods.

23. Raul is going to Egypt next month. He has been looking forward to this vacation all year. Since childhood, Raul has been fascinated with pyramids, especially the Great Pyramid of Giza, which is the oldest of the Seven Wonders of the Ancient World. According to religious custom, Egyptian royalty is buried in the tombs located within the pyramid's great labyrinths. Since it has been many years since Raul read about the pyramid's history, he wants to read a book describing how and why the Egyptians built the Great Pyramid thousands of years ago. Which of the following guides would be the best for Raul?
    a. A Beginner's Guide to Giza, a short book describing the city's best historical sites, published by the Egyptian Tourism Bureau (2015)
    b. The Life of Zahi Hawass, the autobiography of one of Egypt's most famous archaeologists who was one of the first explorers at Giza (2014)
    c. A History of Hieroglyphics, an in-depth look at how archaeologists first broke the ancient code, published by the University of Giza's famed history department (2013)
    d. Who Built the Great Pyramids?, a short summary of the latest research and theories on the ancient Egyptians' religious beliefs and archaeological skills, written by a team of leading experts in the field (2015)

The next five questions are based on the following passage.

Christopher Columbus is often credited for discovering America. This is incorrect. First, it is impossible to "discover" something where people already live; however, Christopher Columbus did explore places in the New World that were previously untouched by Europe, so the term "explorer" would be more accurate. Another correction must be made, as well: Christopher Columbus was not the first European explorer to reach the present day Americas! Rather, it was Leif Erikson who first came to the New World and contacted the natives, nearly five hundred years before Christopher Columbus.

Leif Erikson, the son of Erik the Red (a famous Viking outlaw and explorer in his own right), was born in either 970 or 980, depending on which historian you seek. His own family, though, did not raise Leif, which was a Viking tradition. Instead, one of Erik's prisoners taught Leif reading and writing, languages, sailing, and weaponry. At age 12, Leif was considered a man and returned to his family. He killed a man during a dispute shortly after his return, and the council banished the Erikson clan to Greenland.

In 999, Leif left Greenland and traveled to Norway where he would serve as a guard to King Olaf Tryggvason. It was there that he became a convert to Christianity. Leif later tried to return home with the intention of taking supplies and spreading Christianity to Greenland, however his ship was blown off course and he arrived in a strange new land: present day Newfoundland, Canada.

When he finally returned to his adopted homeland Greenland, Leif consulted with a merchant who had also seen the shores of this previously unknown land we now know as Canada. The son of the legendary Viking explorer then gathered a crew of 35 men and set sail. Leif became the first European to touch foot in the New World as he explored present-day Baffin Island and Labrador, Canada. His crew called the land Vinland since it was plentiful with grapes.

During their time in present-day Newfoundland, Leif's expedition made contact with the natives whom they referred to as Skraelings (which translates to "wretched ones" in Norse). There are several secondhand accounts of their meetings. Some contemporaries described trade between the peoples. Other accounts describe clashes where the Skraelings defeated the Viking explorers with long spears, while still others claim the Vikings dominated the natives. Regardless of the circumstances, it seems that the Vikings made contact of some kind. This happened around 1000, nearly five hundred years before Columbus famously sailed the ocean blue.

Eventually, in 1003, Leif set sail for home and arrived at Greenland with a ship full of timber.

In 1020, seventeen years later, the legendary Viking died. Many believe that Leif Erikson should receive more credit for his contributions in exploring the New World.

24. Which of the following best describes how the author generally presents the information?
    a. Chronological order
    b. Comparison-contrast
    c. Cause-effect
    d. Conclusion-premises

25. Which of the following is an opinion, rather than historical fact, expressed by the author?
    a. Leif Erikson was definitely the son of Erik the Red; however, historians debate the year of his birth.
    b. Leif Erikson's crew called the land Vinland since it was plentiful with grapes.
    c. Leif Erikson deserves more credit for his contributions in exploring the New World.
    d. Leif Erikson explored the Americas nearly five hundred years before Christopher Columbus.

26. Which of the following most accurately describes the author's main conclusion?
    a. Leif Erikson is a legendary Viking explorer.
    b. Leif Erikson deserves more credit for exploring America hundreds of years before Columbus.
    c. Spreading Christianity motivated Leif Erikson's expeditions more than any other factor.
    d. Leif Erikson contacted the natives nearly five hundred years before Columbus.

27. Which of the following best describes the author's intent in the passage?
    a. To entertain
    b. To inform
    c. To alert
    d. To suggest

28. Which of the following can be logically inferred from the passage?
    a. The Vikings disliked exploring the New World.
    b. Leif Erikson's banishment from Iceland led to his exploration of present-day Canada.
    c. Leif Erikson never shared his stories of exploration with the King of Norway.
    d. Historians have difficulty definitively pinpointing events in the Vikings' history.
    The next five questions are based on the chart following a brief introduction to the topic.

The American Civil War was fought from 1861 to 1865. It is the only civil war in American history. While the South's secession was the initiating event of the war, the conflict grew out of several issues like slavery and differing interpretations of individual state rights. General Robert E. Lee led the Confederate Army for the South for the duration of the conflict (although other generals held command positions over individual battles, as you will see below). The North employed a variety of lead generals, but Ulysses S. Grant finished the war as the victorious general. There were more American casualties in the Civil War than any other military conflict in American history.

Civil War Casualties by Battle (approximate)					
Battle	Date	Union General	Confederate General	Union Casualties	Confederate Casualties
Gettysburg	July 1863	George Meade	Robert E. Lee	23,049	28,063
Chancellorsville	May 1863	Joseph Hooker	Robert E. Lee	17,304	13,460
Shiloh	April 1862	Ulysses S. Grant	Albert Sydney Johnston	13,047	10,669
Cold Harbor	May 1864	Ulysses S. Grant	Robert E. Lee	12,737	4,595
Atlanta	July 1864	William T. Sherman	John Bell Hood	3,722	5,500

29. In which of the following battles were there more Confederate casualties than Union casualties?
    a. Cold Harbor
    b. Chancellorsville
    c. Atlanta
    d. Shiloh

30. Which one of the following battles occurred first?
    a. Cold Harbor
    b. Chancellorsville
    c. Atlanta
    d. Shiloh

31. Robert E. Lee did not lead the Confederate forces in which one of the following battles?
    a. Atlanta
    b. Chancellorsville
    c. Cold Harbor
    d. Gettysburg

32. In which of the following battles did the Union casualties exceed the Confederate casualties by the greatest number?
    a. Cold Harbor
    b. Chancellorsville
    c. Atlanta
    d. Shiloh

33. The total number of American casualties suffered at the battle of Gettysburg is about double the total number of casualties suffered at which one of the following battles?
    a. Cold Harbor
    b. Chancellorsville
    c. Atlanta
    d. Shiloh
    The next two questions are based on the graphic that follows a brief introduction to the topic.

The United States Constitution directs Congress to conduct a census of the population to determine the country's population and demographic information. The United States Census Bureau carries out the survey. In 1790, then Secretary of State Thomas Jefferson conducted the first census, and the most recent U.S. census was in 2010. The next U.S. census will be the first to be issued primarily through the Internet.

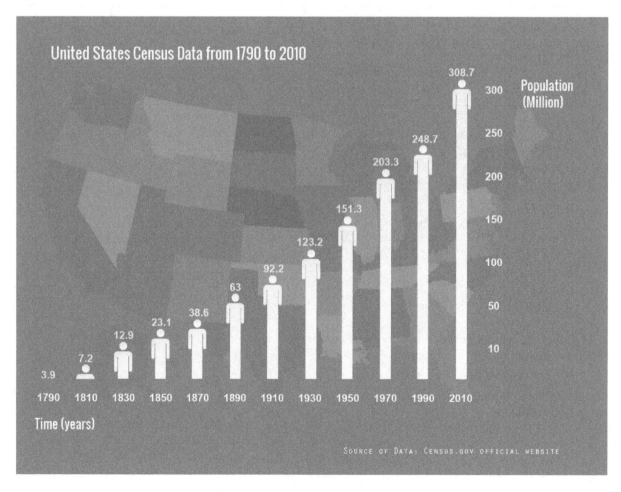

34. In which of the following years was the United States population less than it was in 1930?
    a. 1950
    b. 1970
    c. 1910
    d. 1990

35. In what year did the population increase the most during a twenty-year interval?
    a. From 1930 to 1950
    b. From 1950 to 1970
    c. From 1970 to 1990
    d. From 1990 to 2010

The next question is based on the following outline.

Chapter 5: Outdoor Activities
1. Hiking
        a. Gear
        b. First Aid
2. Camping
        a. Tents & Gear
        b. Camping Activities
3. Cycling
        a. Safety
        b. Finding Cycling Trails
4. Canoeing
        a. Equipment
        b. Tips for Maneuvering

36. What aspect of this outline is inconsistent?
    a. Hiking, which starts with an H, is included with activities that all start with C.
    b. There is no information about gear/equipment for cycling
    c. Rock climbing is not included in the outline.
    d. There is no section for hiking tips.

The next three questions are based on the graphic following a brief introduction to the topic.

A food chain is a diagram used by biologists to better understand ecosystems. It represents the interrelationships between different plants and animals. The energy is derived from the sun and converted into stored energy by plants through photosynthesis, which travels up the food chain. The energy returns to the ecosystem after the organisms die and decompose back into the Earth. This process is an endless cycle.

In food chains, living organisms are grouped into categories called primary producers and consumers, which come in multiple tiers. For example, secondary consumers feed on primary consumers, while tertiary consumers feed on secondary consumers. Apex predators are the animals at the top of the food chain. They are the highest category consumer in an ecosystem, and apex predators do not have natural predators.

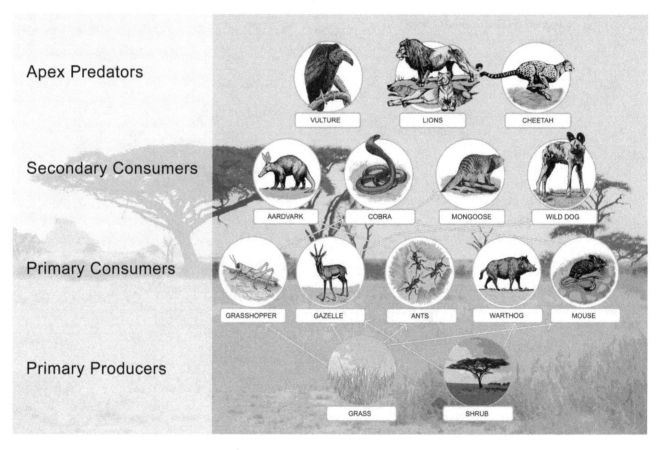

37. Which of the following animals eats primary producers according to the food chain diagram?
    a. Cobra
    b. Gazelle
    c. Wild dog
    d. Aardvark

38. Which of the following animals has no natural predators according to the food chain diagram?
    a. Vulture
    b. Cobra
    c. Mongoose
    d. Aardvark

39. Which of the following is something that the mongoose would eat?
    a. Shrub
    b. Aardvark
    c. Vulture
    d. Mouse

The next four questions are based on the timeline of the life of Alexander Graham Bell.

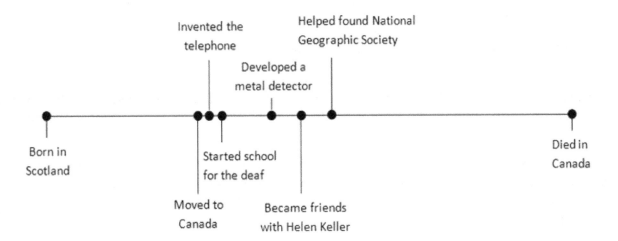

40. Which of the following is the event that occurred fourth on the timeline?
    a. Helped found National Geographic Society
    b. Developed a metal detector
    c. Moved to Canada
    d. Started a school for the deaf

41. Of the pairings in the answer choices, which has the longest gap between the two events?
    a. Moved to Canada and Became friends with Helen Keller
    b. Became friends with Helen Keller and Died in Canada
    c. Started school for the deaf and Developed a metal detector
    d. Born in Scotland and Started school for the deaf

42. Which one of the following statements is accurate based on the timeline?
    a. Bell did nothing significant after he helped found the National Geographic Society.
    b. Bell started a school for the deaf in Canada.
    c. Bell lived in at least two countries.
    d. Developing a metal detector allowed Bell to meet Helen Keller.

43. Which one of the following events occurred most recently?
    a. Bell's invention of the telephone
    b. Bell's founding of the school.
    c. Bell's birth
    d. Bell's move to Canada

44. Which of the following statements would make the best conclusion to an essay about civil rights activist Rosa Parks?

a. On December 1, 1955, Rosa Parks refused to give up her bus seat to a white passenger, setting in motion the Montgomery bus boycott.

b. Rosa Parks was a hero to many, and came to symbolize the way that ordinary people could bring about real change in the Civil Rights Movement.

c. Rosa Parks died in 2005 in Detroit, having moved from Montgomery shortly after the bus boycott.

d. Rosa Parks' arrest was an early part of the Civil Rights Movement, and helped lead to the passage of the Civil Rights Act of 1964.

45. The following exchange occurred after the Baseball Coach's team suffered a heartbreaking loss in the final inning.

Reporter: The team clearly did not rise to the challenge. I'm sure that getting zero hits in twenty at-bats with runners in scoring position hurt the team's chances at winning the game. What are your thoughts on this devastating loss?

Baseball Coach: Hitting with runners in scoring position was not the reason we lost this game. We made numerous errors in the field, and our pitchers gave out too many free passes. Also, we did not even need a hit with runners in scoring position. Many of those at-bats could have driven in the run by simply making contact. Our team did not deserve to win the game.

Which of the following best describes the main point of dispute between the reporter and baseball coach?

a. Whether the loss was heartbreaking.

b. Whether getting zero hits in twenty at-bats with runners in scoring position caused the loss.

c. Numerous errors in the field and pitchers giving too many free passes caused the loss.

d. Whether the team deserved to win the game.

46. Read the following poem. Which option best expresses the symbolic meaning of the "road" and the overall theme?

> Two roads diverged in a yellow wood,
> And sorry I could not travel both
> And be one traveler, long I stood
> And looked down one as far as I could
> To where it bent in the undergrowth;
> Then took the other, as just as fair,
> And having perhaps the better claim,
> Because it was grassy and wanted wear;
> Though as for that the passing there
> Had worn them really about the same,
> And both that morning equally lay
> In leaves no step had trodden black.
> Oh, I kept the first for another day!
> Yet knowing how way leads on to way,
> I doubted if I should ever come back.
> I shall be telling this with a sigh
> Somewhere ages and ages hence:
> Two roads diverged in a wood, and I—
> I took the one less traveled by,
> And that has made all the difference—Robert Frost, "The Road Not Taken"

a. A divergent spot where the traveler had to choose the correct path to his destination
b. A choice between good and evil that the traveler needs to make
c. The traveler's struggle between his lost love and his future prospects
d. Life's journey and the choices with which humans are faced

47. Kimmy is a world famous actress. Millions of people downloaded her leaked movie co-starring her previous boyfriend. Kimmy earns millions through her television show and marketing appearances. There's little wonder that paparazzi track her every move.

What is the argument's primary purpose?
a. Kimmy does not deserve her fame.
b. Kimmy starred in an extremely popular movie.
c. Kimmy earns millions of dollars through her television show and marketing appearances.
d. Kimmy is a highly compensated and extremely popular television and movie actress.

48. Dwight works at a mid-sized regional tech company. He approaches all tasks with unmatched enthusiasm and leads the company in annual sales. The top salesman is always the best employee. Therefore, Dwight is the best employee.

Which of the following most accurately describes how the argument proceeds?
　　a. The argument proceeds by first stating a conclusion and then offering several premises to justify that conclusion.
　　b. The argument proceeds by stating a universal rule and then proceeds to show how this situation is the exception.
　　c. The argument proceeds by stating several facts that serve as the basis for the conclusion at the end of the argument.
　　d. The argument proceeds by stating several facts, offering a universal rule, and then drawing a conclusion by applying the facts to the rule.

Questions 49-51 are based upon the following passage:

This excerpt is adaptation from "The 'Hatchery' of the Sun-Fish"--- *Scientific American*, #711

> I have thought that an example of the intelligence (instinct?) of a class of fish which has come under my observation during my excursions into the Adirondack region of New York State might possibly be of interest to your readers, especially as I am not aware that any one except myself has noticed it, or, at least, has given it publicity.

> The female sun-fish (called, I believe, in England, the roach or bream) makes a "hatchery" for her eggs in this wise. Selecting a spot near the banks of the numerous lakes in which this region abounds, and where the water is about 4 inches deep, and still, she builds, with her tail and snout, a circular embankment 3 inches in height and 2 thick. The circle, which is as perfect a one as could be formed with mathematical instruments, is usually a foot and a half in diameter; and at one side of this circular wall an opening is left by the fish of just sufficient width to admit her body.

> The mother sun-fish, having now built or provided her "hatchery," deposits her spawn within the circular inclosure, and mounts guard at the entrance until the fry are hatched out and are sufficiently large to take charge of themselves. As the embankment, moreover, is built up to the surface of the water, no enemy can very easily obtain an entrance within the inclosure from the top; while there being only one entrance, the fish is able, with comparative ease, to keep out all intruders.

> I have, as I say, noticed this beautiful instinct of the sun-fish for the perpetuity of her species more particularly in the lakes of this region; but doubtless the same habit is common to these fish in other waters.

49. What is the purpose of this passage?
　　a. To show the effects of fish hatcheries on the Adirondack region
　　b. To persuade the audience to study Ichthyology (fish science)
　　c. To depict the sequence of mating among sun-fish
　　d. To enlighten the audience on the habits of sun-fish and their hatcheries

50. What does the word *wise* in this passage most closely mean?
    a. Knowledge
    b. Manner
    c. Shrewd
    d. Ignorance

51. What is the definition of the word *fry* as it appears in the following passage?

    The mother sun-fish, having now built or provided her "hatchery," deposits her spawn within the circular inclosure, and mounts guard at the entrance until the fry are hatched out and are sufficiently large to take charge of themselves.

    a. Fish at the stage of development where they are capable of feeding themselves.
    b. Fish eggs that have been fertilized.
    c. A place where larvae is kept out of danger from other predators.
    d. A dish where fish is placed in oil and fried until golden brown.

52. Read the following passage:

Last week, we adopted a dog from the local animal shelter, after looking for our perfect pet for several months. We wanted a dog that was not too old, but also past the puppy stage, so that training would be less time-intensive and to give an older animal a home. Robin, as she's called, was a perfect match and we filled out our application and upon approval, were permitted to bring her home. Her physical exam and lab work all confirmed she was healthy. We went to the pet store and bought all sorts of bedding, food, toys, and treats to outfit our house as a dog-friendly and fun place. The shelter told us she liked dry food only, which is a relief because wet food is expensive and pretty off-putting. We even got fencing and installed a dog run in the backyard for Robin to roam unattended. Then we took her to the vet to make sure she was healthy. Next week, she starts the dog obedience class that we enrolled her in with a discount coupon from the shelter. It will be a good opportunity to bond with her and establish commands and dominance. When we took her to the park the afternoon after we adopted her, it was clear that she is a sociable and friendly dog, easily playing cohesively with dogs of all sizes and dispositions.

Which of the following is out of sequence in the story?
    a. Last week, we adopted a dog from the local animal shelter, after looking for our perfect pet for several months.
    b. Robin, as she's called, was a perfect match and we filled out our application and upon approval, were permitted to bring her home.
    c. Her physical exam and lab work all confirmed she was healthy.
    d. Next week, she starts the dog obedience class that we enrolled her in with a discount coupon from the shelter.

53. You are a high school math teacher and one of your students, Marcus, emailed asking to come see you after the latest exam. His email said he was disappointed and surprised with his grade and wanted to inquire about extra credit work to recoup points he lost on the exam. You decided to look over the details of his performance in your course to find any potential causes for his poor marks and to offer him informed tips to improve for the next exam. Thankfully, you keep detailed records to tracks each student's grades. You have four pieces of information to evaluate before he comes in to meet with you: a graph of his scores on the four exams he's taken so far, a graph of the number of absences he's had each week thus far in the course, a graph of the percentage of homework assignments he's completed each week, and an email from his basketball coach.

From: William Cooper, Boys Varsity Basketball Coach
To: All academic teachers
Re: Marco

Marco will be competing in the Northeast Regional Basketball tournament next week and will be absent from classes Tuesday through Friday. The student athletes will be responsible for obtaining their assignments and making arrangements to complete any missed material. If you have any questions, please don't hesitate to reach out to me. While I understand that this is not ideal so close to final exams, but this is the first time our Ravens have made it so far in the tournament and we are excited to see how well they will perform.

Thanks,
Coach William Cooper

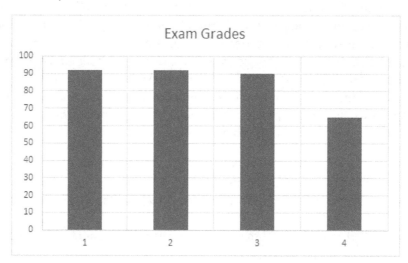

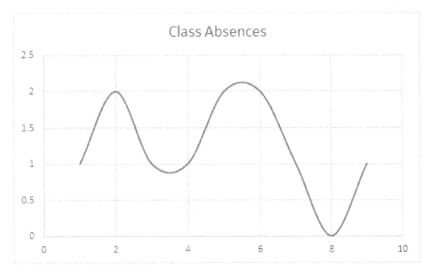

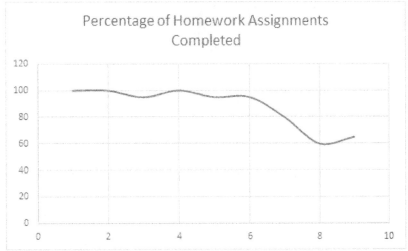

Which of the given information sources provides a possible explanation for a Marco's recent poor exam grade?

    a. The email from his basketball coach about the tournament

    b. The graph of his exam marks

    c. The graph of his class absences each week

    d. The graph of the percentage of homework assignments completed

Mathematics

1. Which of the following numbers has the greatest value?

    a. 1.4378

    b. 1.07548

    c. 1.43592

    d. 0.89409

2. The value of 6 x 12 is the same as:
   a. 2 x 4 x 4 x 2
   b. 7 x 4 x 3
   c. 6 x 6 x 3
   d. 3 x 3 x 4 x 2

3. This chart indicates how many sales of CDs, vinyl records, and MP3 downloads occurred over the last year. Approximately what percentage of the total sales was from CDs?

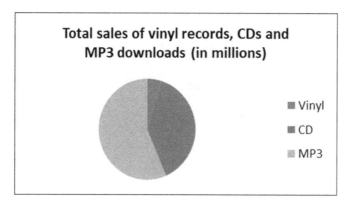

   a. 55%
   b. 25%
   c. 40%
   d. 5%

4. After a 20% sale discount, Frank purchased a new refrigerator for $850. How much did he save from the original price?
   a. $170
   b. $212.50
   c. $105.75
   d. $200

5. Which of the following is largest?
   a. 0.45
   b. 0.096
   c. 0.3
   d. 0.313

6. What is the value of b in this equation?
$$5b - 4 = 2b + 17$$

   a. 13
   b. 24
   c. 7
   d. 21

7. A school has 15 teachers and 20 teaching assistants. They have 200 students. What is the ratio of faculty to students?

    a. 3:20

    b. 4:17

    c. 3:2

    d. 7:40

8. Express the solution to the following problem in decimal form:

$$\frac{3}{5} \times \frac{7}{10} \div \frac{1}{2}$$

    a. 0.042

    b. 84%

    c. 0.84

    d. 0.42

9. A student gets an 85% on a test with 20 questions. How many answers did the student solve correctly?

    a. 15

    b. 16

    c. 17

    d. 18

10. If Sarah reads at an average rate of 21 pages in four nights, how long will it take her to read 140 pages?

    a. 6 nights

    b. 26 nights

    c. 8 nights

    d. 27 nights

11. Alan currently weighs 200 pounds, but he wants to lose weight to get down to 175 pounds. What is this difference in kilograms? (1 pound is approximately equal to 0.45 kilograms.)

    a. 9 kg

    b. 11.25 kg

    c. 78.75 kg

    d. 90 kg

12. Johnny earns $2334.50 from his job each month. He pays $1437 for monthly expenses. Johnny is planning a vacation in 3 months' time that he estimates will cost $1750 total. How much will Johnny have left over from three months' of saving once he pays for his vacation?

    a. $948.50

    b. $584.50

    c. $852.50

    d. $942.50

13. What is $\frac{420}{98}$ rounded to the nearest integer?
    a. 3
    b. 4
    c. 5
    d. 6

14. Solve the following:

$$4 \times 7 + (25 - 21)^2 \div 2$$

    a. 512
    b. 36
    c. 60.5
    d. 22

15. The total perimeter of a rectangle is 36 cm. If the length of each side is 12 cm, what is the width?
    a. 3 cm
    b. 12 cm
    c. 6 cm
    d. 8 cm

16. Dwayne has received the following scores on his math tests: 78, 92, 83, 97. What score must Dwayne get on his next math test to have an overall average of at least 90?
    a. 89
    b. 98
    c. 95
    d. 100

17. What is the overall median of Dwayne's current scores: 78, 92, 83, 97?
    a. 19
    b. 85
    c. 83
    d. 87.5

18. Solve the following:

$$\left(\sqrt{36} \times \sqrt{16}\right) - 3^2$$

    a. 30
    b. 21
    c. 15
    d. 13

19. In Jim's school, there are 3 girls for every 2 boys. There are 650 students in total. Using this information, how many students are girls?
    a. 260
    b. 130
    c. 65
    d. 390

20. What is the solution to 4 x 7 + $(25 - 21)^2 \div 2$?
   a. 512
   b. 36
   c. 60.5
   d. 22

21. Kimberley earns $10 an hour babysitting, and after 10 p.m., she earns $12 an hour, with the amount paid being rounded to the nearest hour accordingly. On her last job, she worked from 5:30 p.m. to 11 p.m. In total, how much did Kimberley earn on her last job?
   a. $45
   b. $57
   c. $62
   d. $42

22. Solve this equation:

$$9x + x - 7 = 16 + 2x$$

   a. -4

   b. 3

   c. $\frac{9}{8}$

   d. $\frac{23}{8}$

23. Arrange the following numbers from least to greatest value:
   $0.85, \frac{4}{5}, \frac{2}{3}, \frac{91}{100}$

   a. $0.85, \frac{4}{5}, \frac{2}{3}, \frac{91}{100}$

   b. $\frac{4}{5}, 0.85, \frac{91}{100}, \frac{2}{3}$

   c. $\frac{2}{3}, \frac{4}{5}, 0.85, \frac{91}{100}$

   d. $0.85, \frac{91}{100}, \frac{4}{5}, \frac{2}{3}$

24. Keith's bakery had 252 customers go through its doors last week. This week, that number increased to 378. Express this increase as a percentage.
   a. 26%
   b. 50%
   c. 35%
   d. 12%

25. If $4x - 3 = 5$, then $x =$
   a. 1
   b. 2
   c. 3
   d. 4

26. Simplify the following fraction:

$$\frac{\frac{5}{7}}{\frac{9}{11}}$$

    a. $\frac{55}{63}$

    b. $\frac{7}{1000}$

    c. $\frac{13}{15}$

    d. $\frac{5}{11}$

27. The following graph compares the various test scores of the top three students in each of these teacher's classes. Based on the graph, which teacher's students had the lowest range of test scores?

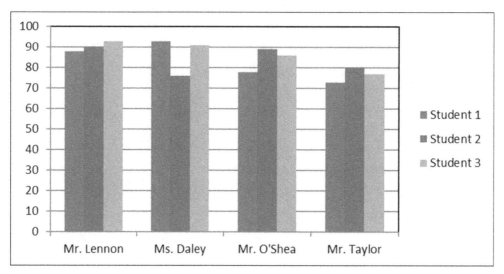

    a. Mr. Lennon
    b. Mr. O'Shea
    c. Mr. Taylor
    d. Ms. Daley

28. Bernard can make $80 per day. If he needs to make $300 and only works full days, how many days will this take?
    a. 2
    b. 3
    c. 4
    d. 5

29. Using the following diagram, calculate the total circumference, rounding to the nearest decimal place:

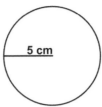

5 cm

    a. 25.0 cm
    b. 15.7 cm
    c. 78.5 cm
    d. 31.4 cm

30. Which measure for the center of a small sample set would be most affected by outliers?
    a. Mean
    b. Median
    c. Mode
    d. None of the above

31. A line that travels from the bottom-left of a graph to the upper-right of the graph indicates what kind of relationship between a predictor and a dependent variable?
    a. Positive
    b. Negative
    c. Exponential
    d. Logarithmic

32. How many kilometers is 4382 feet?
    a. 1.336 kilometers
    b. 14,376 kilometers
    c. 1.437 kilometers
    d. 13,336 kilometers

33. Which of the following is the best description of the relationship between Y and X?
    a. The data has normal distribution.
    b. X and Y have a negative relationship.
    c. No relationship
    d. X and Y have a positive relationship.

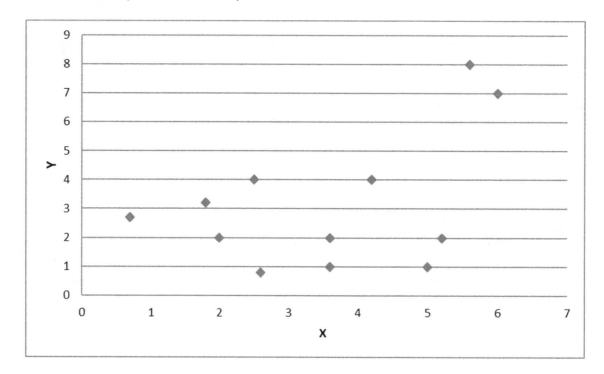

34. What is the slope of this line?

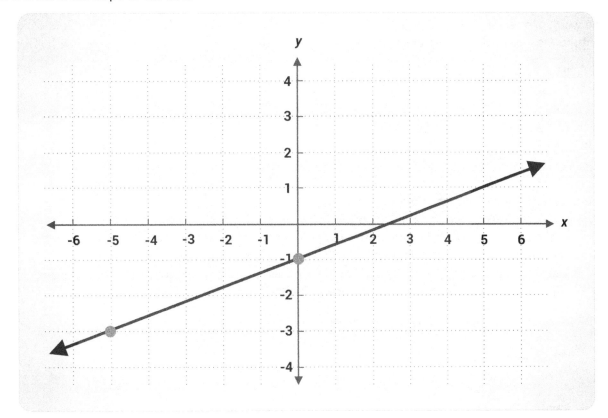

    a. 2

    b. $\frac{5}{2}$

    c. $\frac{1}{2}$

    d. $\frac{2}{5}$

35. What is the perimeter of the figure below? Note that the solid outer line is the perimeter.

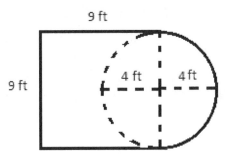

    a. 48.565 ft
    b. 39.565 ft
    c. 19.78 ft
    d. 30.565 ft

36. Which of the following equations best represents the problem below?

The width of a rectangle is 2 centimeters less than the length. If the perimeter of the rectangle is 44 centimeters, then what are the dimensions of the rectangle?

   a. $2l + 2(l - 2) = 44$
   b. $l + 2) + (l + 2) + l = 48$
   c. $l \times (l - 2) = 44$
   d. $(l + 2) + (l + 2) + l = 44$

Science

1. Which statement about white blood cells is true?
   a. B cells are responsible for antibody production.
   b. White blood cells are made in the white/yellow cartilage before they enter the bloodstream.
   c. Platelets, a special class of white blood cell, function to clot blood and stop bleeding.
   d. The majority of white blood cells only activate during the age of puberty, which explains why children and the elderly are particularly susceptible to disease.

2. Which locations in the digestive system are sites of chemical digestion?
     I. Mouth
     II. Stomach
     III. Small Intestine

   a. II only
   b. III only
   c. II and III only
   d. I, II, and III

3. Which of the following are functions of the urinary system?
     I. Synthesizing calcitriol and secreting erythropoietin
     II. Regulating the concentrations of sodium, potassium, chloride, calcium, and other ions
     III. Reabsorbing or secreting hydrogen ions and bicarbonate
     IV. Detecting reductions in blood volume and pressure

   a. I, II, and III
   b. II and III
   c. II, III, and IV
   d. All of the above

4. Which of the following structures is unique to eukaryotic cells?
   a. Cell walls
   b. Nucleuses
   c. Cell membranes
   d. Vacuoles

5. Which is the cellular organelle used for digestion to recycle materials?
   a. The Golgi apparatus
   b. The lysosome
   c. The centrioles
   d. The mitochondria

6. A rock has a mass of 14.3 grams (g) and a volume of 5.4 cm^3, what is its density?
   a. 8.90 g/cm^3
   b. 0.38 g/cm^3
   c. 77.22 g/cm^3
   d. 2.65 g/cm^3

7. Why do arteries have valves?
   a. They have valves to maintain high blood pressure so that capillaries diffuse nutrients properly.
   b. Their valves are designed to prevent backflow due to their low blood pressure.
   c. They have valves due to a leftover trait from evolution that, like the appendix, are useless.
   d. They do not have valves, but veins do.

8. If the pressure in the pulmonary artery is increased above normal, which chamber of the heart will be affected first?
   a. The right atrium
   b. The left atrium
   c. The right ventricle
   d. The left ventricle

9. What is the purpose of sodium bicarbonate when released into the lumen of the small intestine?
   a. It works to chemically digest fats in the chyme.
   b. It decreases the pH of the chyme so as to prevent harm to the intestine.
   c. It works to chemically digest proteins in the chyme.
   d. It increases the pH of the chyme so as to prevent harm to the intestine.

10. Which of the following describes a reflex arc?
    a. The storage and recall of memory
    b. The maintenance of visual and auditory acuity
    c. The autoregulation of heart rate and blood pressure
    d. A stimulus and response controlled by the spinal cord

11. Describe the synthesis of the lagging strand of DNA.
    a. DNA polymerases synthesize DNA continuously after initially attaching to a primase.
    b. DNA polymerases synthesize DNA discontinuously in pieces called Okazaki fragments after initially attaching to primases.
    c. DNA polymerases synthesize DNA discontinuously in pieces called Okazaki fragments after initially attaching to RNA primers.
    d. DNA polymerases synthesize DNA discontinuously in pieces called Okazaki fragments which are joined together in the end by a DNA helicase.

12. Using anatomical terms, what is the relationship of the sternum relative to the deltoid?
    a. Medial
    b. Lateral
    c. Superficial
    d. Posterior

13. Ligaments connect what?
    a. Muscle to muscle
    b. Bone to bone
    c. Bone to muscle
    d. Muscle to tendon

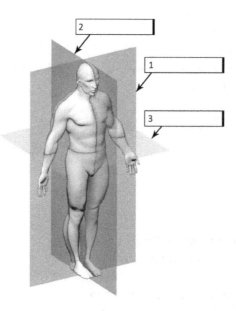

14. Identify the correct sequence of the 3 primary body planes as numbered 1, 2, and 3 in the above image.
    a. Plane 1 is coronal, plane 2 is sagittal, and plane 3 is transverse.
    b. Plane 1 is sagittal, plane 2 is coronal, and plane 3 is medial.
    c. Plane 1 is coronal, plane 2 is sagittal, and plane 3 is medial.
    d. Plane 1 is sagittal, plane 2 is coronal, and plane 3 is transverse.

15. Which of the following is NOT a major function of the respiratory system in humans?
    a. It provides a large surface area for gas exchange of oxygen and carbon dioxide.
    b. It helps regulate the blood's pH.
    c. It helps cushion the heart against jarring motions.
    d. It is responsible for vocalization.

16. Which of the following is NOT a function of the forebrain?
    a. To regulate blood pressure and heart rate
    b. To perceive and interpret emotional responses like fear and anger
    c. To perceive and interpret visual input from the eyes
    d. To integrate voluntary movement

17. What is the major difference between somatic and germline mutations?
   a. Somatic mutations usually benefit the individual while germline mutations usually harm them.
   b. Since germline mutations only affect one cell, they are less noticeable than the rapidly dividing somatic cells.
   c. Somatic mutations are not expressed for several generations, but germline mutations are expressed immediately.
   d. Germline mutations are usually inherited while somatic mutations will affect only the individual.

18. A child complains of heavy breathing even when relaxing. They are an otherwise healthy child with no history of respiratory problems. What might be the issue?
   a. Asthma
   b. Blood clot
   c. Hyperventilation
   d. Exercising too hard

19. Find the lowest coefficients that will balance the following combustion equation.

$$\_\_C_2H_{10}+\_\_O_2 \rightarrow \_\_H_2O+\_\_CO_2$$

   a. 1:5:5:2
   b. 4:10:20:8
   c. 2:9:10:4
   d. 2:5:10:4

20. What is the purpose of a catalyst?
   a. To increase a reaction rate by increasing the activation energy
   b. To increase a reaction's rate by increasing the temperature
   c. To increase a reaction's rate by decreasing the activation energy
   d. To increase a reaction's rate by decreasing the temperature

21. Most catalysts found in biological systems are which of the following?
   a. Special lipids called cofactors.
   b. Special proteins called enzymes.
   c. Special lipids called enzymes.
   d. Special proteins called cofactors.

22. Which statement is true about the pH of a solution?
   a. A solution cannot have a pH less than 1.
   b. The more hydroxide ions in the solution, the higher the pH.
   c. If an acid has a pH of greater than 2, it is considered a weak base.
   d. A solution with a pH of 2 has ten times the amount of hydrogen ions than a solution with a power of 1.

23. Salts like sodium iodide (NaI) and potassium chloride (KCl) use what type of bond?
   a. Ionic bonds
   b. Disulfide bridges
   c. Covalent bonds
   d. London dispersion forces

24. Which of the following is unique to covalent bonds?
    a. Most covalent bonds are formed between the elements H, F, N, and O.
    b. Covalent bonds are dependent on forming dipoles.
    c. Bonding electrons are shared between two or more atoms.
    d. Molecules with covalent bonds tend to have a crystalline solid structure.

25. Which of the following describes a typical gas?
    a. Indefinite shape and indefinite volume
    b. Indefinite shape and definite volume
    c. Definite shape and definite volume
    d. Definite shape and indefinite volume

26. Which of the following areas of the body has the most sweat glands?
    a. Upper back
    b. Arms
    c. Feet
    d. Palms

27. A patient's body is not properly filtering blood. Which of the following body parts is most likely malfunctioning?
    a. Medulla
    B. Heart
    C. Nephrons
    D. Renal cortex

28. A pediatrician notes that an infant's cartilage is disappearing and being replaced by bone. What process has the doctor observed?
    a. Mineralization
    b. Ossification
    c. Osteoporosis
    d. Calcification

29. The epidermis is composed of what type of cells?
    a. Osteoclasts
    b. Connective
    c. Dendritic
    d. Epithelial

30. Which of the following is directly transcribed from DNA and represents the first step in protein building?
    a. siRNA
    b. rRNA
    c. mRNA
    d. tRNA

31. What information does a genotype give that a phenotype does not?
    a. The genotype necessarily includes the proteins coded for by its alleles.
    b. The genotype will always show an organism's recessive alleles.
    c. The genotype must include the organism's physical characteristics.
    d. The genotype shows what an organism's parents looked like.

	T	t
T		
t		

32. Which statement is supported by the Punnett square above, if "T" = Tall and "t" = short?
    a. Both parents are homozygous tall.
    b. 100% of the offspring will be tall because both parents are tall.
    c. There is a 25% chance that an offspring will be short.
    d. The short allele will soon die out.

33. Which of the following is a chief difference between evaporation and boiling?
    a. Liquids boil only at the surface while they evaporate equally throughout the liquid.
    b. Evaporating substances change from gas to liquid while boiling substances change from liquid to gas.
    c. Evaporation happens in nature while boiling is a manmade phenomenon.
    d. Evaporation can happen below a liquid's boiling point.

34. Which of the following CANNOT be found in a human cell's genes?
    a. Sequences of amino acids to be transcribed into mRNA
    b. Lethal recessive traits like sickle cell anemia
    c. Mutated DNA
    d. DNA that codes for proteins the cell doesn't use

35. Which of the following is a special property of water?
    a. Water easily flows through phospholipid bilayers.
    b. A water molecule's oxygen atom allows fish to breathe.
    c. Water is highly cohesive which explains its high melting point.
    d. Water can self-hydrolyze and decompose into hydrogen and oxygen.

36. What is an isotope? For any given element, it is an atom with which of the following?
    a. a different atomic number.
    b. a different number of protons.
    c. a different number of electrons.
    d. a different mass number.

37. What is the electrical charge of the nucleus?
   a. A nucleus always has a positive charge.
   b. A stable nucleus has a positive charge, but a radioactive nucleus may have no charge and instead be neutral.
   c. A nucleus always has no charge and is instead neutral.
   d. A stable nucleus has no charge and is instead neutral, but a radioactive nucleus may have a charge.

38. A student believes that there is an inverse relationship between sugar consumption and test scores. To test this hypothesis, he recruits several people to eat sugar, wait one hour, and take a short aptitude test afterwards. The student will compile the participants' sugar intake levels and test scores. How should the student conduct the experiment?
   a. One round of testing, where each participant consumes a different level of sugar.
   b. Two rounds of testing: The first, where each participant consumes a different level of sugar, and the second, where each participant consumes the same level as they did in Round 1.
   c. Two rounds of testing: The first, where each participant consumes the same level of sugar as each other, and the second, where each participant consumes the same level of sugar as each other but at higher levels than in Round 1.
   d. One round of testing, where each participant consumes the same level of sugar.

39. Which of the following creates sperm?
   a. Prostate gland
   b. Seminal vesicles
   c. Scrotum
   d. Seminiferous tubules

40. A researcher is exploring factors that contribute to the GPA of college students. While the sample is small, the researcher is trying to determine what the data shows. What can be reasoned from the table below?

Student	Maintains a Calendar?	Takes Notes?	GPA
A	sometimes	often	3.1
B	never	always	3.9
C	never	never	2.0
D	sometimes	often	2.7

   a. No college students consistently maintain a calendar of events.
   b. There is an inverse correlation between maintaining a calendar and GPA, and there is a positive correlation between taking notes and GPA.
   c. There is a positive correlation between maintaining a calendar and GPA, and there is no correlation between taking notes and GPA.
   d. There is no correlation between maintaining a calendar and GPA, and there is a positive correlation between taking notes and GPA.

41. Four different groups of the same species of peas are grown and exposed to differing levels of sunlight, water, and fertilizer as documented in the table below. The data in the water and fertilizer columns indicates how many times the peas are watered or fertilized per week, respectively. Group 2 is the only group that withered. What is a reasonable explanation for this occurrence?

Group	Sunlight	Water	Fertilizer
1	partial sun	4 mL/hr	1
2	full sun	7 mL/hr	1
3	no sun	14 mL/hr	2
4	partial sun	3 mL/hr	2

    a. Insects gnawed away the stem of the plant.
    b. The roots rotted due to poor drainage.
    c. The soil type had nutrition deficiencies.
    d. This species of peas does not thrive in full sunlight.

42. Which of the following functions corresponds to the parasympathetic nervous system?
    a. It stimulates the fight-or-flight response.
    b. It increases heart rate.
    c. It stimulates digestion.
    d. It increases bronchiole dilation.

43. According to the periodic table, which of the following elements is the least reactive?
    a. Fluorine
    b. Silicon
    c. Neon
    d. Gallium

44. The Human Genome Project is a worldwide research project launched in 1990 to map the entire human genome. Although the Project was faced with the monumental challenge of analyzing tons and tons of data, its objective was completed in 2003 and ahead of its deadline by two years. Which of the following inventions likely had the greatest impact on this project?
    a. The sonogram
    b. X-ray diffraction
    c. The microprocessor
    d. Magnetic Resonance Imaging (MRI)

45. Which of the following inventions likely had the greatest improvement on the ability to combat nutrition deficiencies in developing countries?
    a. Food products fortified with dietary vitamins and minerals
    b. Integrated statistical models of fish populations
    c. Advances so that microscopes can use thicker tissue samples
    d. Refrigerated train cars for transportation of food

46. Which of the following is the gland that helps regulate calcium levels?
    a. Osteotoid gland
    b. Pineal gland
    c. Parathyroid glands
    d. Thymus gland

47. Anya was paid by Company X to analyze dwindling honeybee populations of the Southwest. After measuring hive populations over several months, she noticed no patterns in the geographic distributions of the deaths after comparisons with local maps of interest. This supported her hypothesis, so she took samples of the honey and the bees from the hives and performed dozens of dissections to confirm her suspicions. Which of the following is the most likely hypothesis upon which this research was performed?
    a. Honeybees are being killed off and their hives destroyed by other extremely aggressive species of bees from the South.
    b. Honeybees are contracting parasites in large droves.
    c. Honeybees are so sensitive to certain pesticides that they die on contact.
    d. Honeybees die in larger numbers around cell phone towers.

48. Explain the Law of Conservation of Mass as it applies to this reaction: 2H2 + O2 ➜ 2H2O.
    a. Electrons are lost.
    b. The hydrogen loses mass.
    c. New oxygen atoms are formed.
    d. There is no decrease or increase of matter

49. Which of the following is the best unit to measure the amount of blood in the human body?
    a. Ounces
    b. Liters
    c. Milliliters
    d. Pounds

50. Which of the following systems does not include a transportation system throughout the body?
    a. Cardiovascular system
    b. Endocrine system
    c. Immune system
    d. Nervous system

51. Which of the following correctly identifies a difference between the primary and secondary immune response?
    a. In the secondary response, macrophages migrate to the lymph nodes to present the foreign microorganism to helped T lymphocytes.
    b. The humeral immunity that characterizes the primary response is coordinated by T lymphocytes.
    c. The primary response is quicker and more powerful than the secondary response.
    d. Suppressor T cells activate in the secondary response to prevent an overactive immune response.

52. Eosinophils are best described as which of the following?
    a. A type of granulocyte that secretes histamine, which stimulates the inflammatory response.
    b. The most abundant type of white blood cell and they secrete substances that are toxic to pathogens.
    c. A type of granulocyte found under mucous membranes and defends against multicellular parasites.

d. A type of circulating granulocyte that is aggressive and has high phagocytic activity.

53. Which of the following correctly matches a category of protein with a physiologic example?
    a. Keratin is a structural protein
    b. Antigens are hormonal proteins
    c. Channel proteins are marker proteins
    d. Actin is a transport protein

English and Language Usage

1. Which of the following sentences has an error in capitalization?
    a. The East Coast has experienced very unpredictable weather this year.
    b. My Uncle owns a home in Florida, where he lives in the winter.
    c. I am taking English Composition II on campus this fall.
    d. There are several nice beaches we can visit on our trip to the Jersey Shore this summer.

2. Julia Robinson, an avid photographer in her spare time, was able to capture stunning shots of the local wildlife on her last business trip to Australia.
Which of the following is an adjective in the preceding sentence?
    a. Time
    b. Capture
    c. Avid
    d. Photographer

3. Which of the following sentences uses correct punctuation?
    a. Carole is not currently working; her focus is on her children at the moment.
    b. Carole is not currently working and her focus is on her children at the moment.
    c. Carole is not currently working, her focus is on her children at the moment.
    d. Carole is not currently working her focus is on her children at the moment.

4. Which of these examples is a compound sentence?
    a. Alex and Shane spent the morning coloring and later took a walk down to the park.
    b. After coloring all morning, Alex and Shane spent the afternoon at the park.
    c. Alex and Shane spent the morning coloring, and then they took a walk down to the park.
    d. After coloring all morning and spending part of the day at the park, Alex and Shane took a nap.

5. Which of these examples shows incorrect use of subject-verb agreement?
    a. Neither of the cars are parked on the street.
    b. Both of my kids are going to camp this summer.
    c. Any of your friends are welcome to join us on the trip in November.
    d. Each of the clothing options is appropriate for the job interview.

6. When it gets warm in the spring, _____ and _____ like to go fishing at Cobbs Creek.
Which of the following word pairs should be used in the blanks above?
    a. me, him
    b. he, I
    c. him, I
    d. he, me

7. Which example shows correct comma usage for dates?
   a. The due date for the final paper in the course is Monday, May 16, 2016.
   b. The due date for the final paper in the course is Monday, May 16 2016.
   c. The due date for the final project in the course is Monday, May, 16, 2016.
   d. The due date for the final project in the course is Monday May 16, 2016.

8. Which of the following uses correct spelling?
   a. Leslie knew that training for the Philadelphia Marathon would take dicsipline and perserverance, but she was up to the challenge.
   b. Leslie knew that training for the Philadelphia Marathon would take discipline and perseverence, but she was up to the challenge.
   c. Leslie knew that training for the Philadelphia Marathon would take disiplin and perservearance, but she was up to the challenge.
   d. Leslie knew that training for the Philadelphia Marathon would take discipline and perseverance, but she was up to the challenge.

9. At last night's company function, in honor of Mr. Robertson's retirement, several employees spoke kindly about his career achievements.

In the preceding sentence, what part of speech is the word *function*?
   a. Adjective
   b. Adverb
   c. Verb
   d. Noun

10. Which of the examples uses the correct plural form?
    a. Tomatos
    b. Analysis
    c. Cacti
    d. Criterion

11. Which of the following examples uses correct punctuation?
    a. The moderator asked the candidates, "Is each of you prepared to discuss your position on global warming?".
    b. The moderator asked the candidates, "Is each of you prepared to discuss your position on global warming?"
    c. The moderator asked the candidates, 'Is each of you prepared to discuss your position on global warming?'
    d. The moderator asked the candidates, "Is each of you prepared to discuss your position on global warming"?

12. Based on the words *transfer, transact, translation, transport,* what is the meaning of the prefix *trans*?
    a. Separation
    b. All, everywhere
    c. Forward
    d. Across, beyond, over

13. In which of the following sentences does the word *part* function as an adjective?
    a. The part Brian was asked to play required many hours of research.
    b. She parts ways with the woodsman at the end of the book.
    c. The entire team played a part in the success of the project.
    d. Ronaldo is part Irish on his mother's side of the family.

14. All of Shannon's family and friends helped her to celebrate her 50th birthday at Café Sorrento. Which of the following is the complete subject of the preceding sentence?
    a. Family and friends
    b. All
    c. All of Shannon's family and friends
    d. Shannon's family and friends

15. Which of the following sentences uses second person point of view?
    a. I don't want to make plans for the weekend before I see my work schedule.
    b. She had to miss the last three yoga classes due to illness.
    c. Pluto is no longer considered a planet because it is not gravitationally dominant.
    d. Be sure to turn off all of the lights before locking up for the night.

16. As the tour group approached the bottom of Chichen Itza, the prodigious Mayan pyramid, they became nervous about climbing its distant peak.

Based on the context of the sentence, which of the following words shows the correct meaning of the word *prodigious*?
    a. Very large
    b. Famous
    c. Very old
    d. Fancy

17. Which of the following sentences correctly uses a hyphen?
    a. Last-year, many of the players felt unsure of the coach's methods.
    b. Some of the furniture she selected seemed a bit over - the - top for the space.
    c. Henry is a beagle-mix and is ready for adoption this weekend.
    d. Geena works to maintain a good relationship with her ex-husband to the benefit of their children.

18. Which of the following examples correctly uses quotation marks?
    a. "Where the Red Fern Grows" was one of my favorite novels as a child.
    b. Though he is famous for his roles in films like "The Great Gatsby" and "Titanic," Leonardo DiCaprio has never won an Oscar.
    c. Sylvia Plath's poem, "Daddy" will be the subject of this week's group discussion.
    d. "The New York Times" reported that many fans are disappointed in some of the trades made by the Yankees this off-season.

19. Which of the following sentences shows correct word usage?
    a. It's often been said that work is better then rest.
    b. Its often been said that work is better then rest.
    c. It's often been said that work is better than rest.
    d. Its often been said that work is better than rest.

20. Glorify, fortify, gentrify, acidify

Based on the preceding words, what is the correct meaning of the suffix –fy?
   a. Marked by, given to
   b. Doer, believer
   c. Make, cause, cause to have
   d. Process, state, rank

21. Which of the following uses correct spelling?
   a. Jed was disatisfied with the acommodations at his hotel, so he requested another room.
   b. Jed was dissatisfied with the accommodations at his hotel, so he requested another room.
   c. Jed was dissatisfied with the accomodations at his hotel, so he requested another room.
   d. Jed was disatisfied with the accommodations at his hotel, so he requested another room.

22. Which of the following is an imperative sentence?
   a. Pennsylvania's state flag includes two draft horses and an eagle.
   b. Go down to the basement and check the hot water heater for signs of a leak.
   c. You must be so excited to have a new baby on the way!
   d. How many countries speak Spanish?

23. After a long day at work, Tracy had dinner with her family, and then took a walk to the park.
What are the transitional words in the preceding sentence?
   a. After, then
   b. At, with, to
   c. Had, took
   d. A, the

24. Which of the following examples is a compound sentence?
   a. Shawn and Jerome played soccer in the backyard for two hours.
   b. Marissa last saw Elena and talked to her this morning.
   c. The baby was sick, so I decided to stay home from work.
   d. Denise, Kurt, and Eric went for a run after dinner.

25. Robert needed to find at least four sources for his final project, so he searched several library databases for reliable academic research.
Which words function as nouns in the preceding sentence?
   a. Robert, sources, project, databases, research
   b. Robert, sources, final, project, databases, academic, research
   c. Robert, sources, project, he, library, databases, research
   d. Sources, project, databases, research

26. Which of the following sentences uses correct subject-verb agreement?
   a. There is two constellations that can be seen from the back of the house.
   b. At least four of the sheep needs to be sheared before the end of summer.
   c. Lots of people were auditioning for the singing competition on Saturday.
   d. Everyone in the group have completed the assignment on time.

27. Philadelphia is home to some excellent walking tours where visitors can learn more about the culture and rich history of the city of brotherly love.
What are the adjectives in the preceding sentence?
  a. Philadelphia, tours, visitors, culture, history, city, love
  b. Excellent, walking, rich, brotherly
  c. Is, can, learn
  d. To, about, of

28. The realtor showed _____ and _____ a house on Wednesday afternoon.
Which of the following pronoun pairs should be used in the blanks above?
  a. She, I
  b. She, me
  c. Me, her
  d. Her, me

29. Which of the following examples uses correct punctuation?
  a. Recommended supplies for the hunting trip include the following: rain gear, large backpack, hiking boots, flashlight, and non-perishable foods.
  b. I left the store, because I forgot my wallet.
  c. As soon as the team checked into the hotel; they met in the lobby for a group photo.
  d. None of the furniture came in on time: so they weren't able to move in to the new apartment.

30. Which of the following sentences shows correct word usage?
  a. Your going to have to put you're jacket over their.
  b. You're going to have to put your jacket over there.
  c. Your going to have to put you're jacket over they're.
  d. You're going to have to put you're jacket over their.

31. A student wants to rewrite the following sentence:
    Entrepreneurs use their ideas to make money.

He wants to use the word *money* as a verb, but he isn't sure which word ending to use. What is the appropriate suffix to add to *money* to complete the following sentence?

                    Entrepreneurs _____ their ideas.

  a. –ize
  b. –ical
  c. –en
  d. –ful

32. A teacher notices that, when students are talking to each other between classes, they are using their own unique vocabulary words and expressions to talk about their daily lives. When the teacher hears these non-standard words that are specific to one age or cultural group, what type of language is she listening to?
  a. Slang
  b. Jargon
  c. Dialect
  d. Vernacular

33. A teacher wants to counsel a student about using the word *ain't* in a research paper for a high school English class. What advice should the teacher give?

    a. *Ain't* is not in the dictionary, so it isn't a word.

    b. Because the student isn't in college yet, *ain't* is an appropriate expression for a high school writer.

    c. *Ain't* is incorrect English and should not be part of a serious student's vocabulary because it sounds uneducated.

    d. *Ain't* is a colloquial expression, and while it may be appropriate in a conversational setting, it is not standard in academic writing.

Answer Explanations

Reading

1. B: To *propagate* means to spread, disseminate, promote, or otherwise make known an idea, thought, or belief. Xavier is clearly communicating his belief in dragons to his friends. Choices A and D, *whispered* and *shouted*, denote a lowered and raised decibel, respectively. Choice C, *persuaded*, means to cause someone to believe something in a convincing fashion. Although *persuaded* is a better answer than *whispered* or *shouted*, *expressed* is the best answer because *express* means to convey or communicate information. Choice B is the correct answer.

2. D: We are looking for the claim that is least supportive of the argument that the American economy is healthy. Choice A says that the GDP increased by 2% last year, which supports a claim of health. Choice B relays that unemployment is the lowest it's been in over a decade, a sign of a strong economy. Choice C states that average household income is at a historical high point. In contrast, the final choice draws a negative conclusion about the economy—a decrease in output even after investments—therefore, a declining manufacturing sector is least supportive that the economy is healthy. Choice D is the correct answer.

3. C: The question tells us that Noam Chomsky is a linguist, philosopher, social scientist, cognitive scientist, historian, social critic, and political activist. Choice A lists section 700, arts and recreation, which is not relevant. Choice B lists section 800, literature, which does not correspond to the answer. Choice D lists 200, religion, which is not applicable. Thus, Choice C is the correct answer since 100, 400, and 900 are areas of Chomsky's expertise: philosophy, languages, and history.

4. C: This question is asking you the best section to find information about anarchism. Choice A is not relevant. Anarchism is not a religion, so Choice B is not appropriate. Choice D would include history and perhaps provide some appropriate resources. However, anarchism is by nature and definition a social science; therefore, it best fits within the social science section. The correct section is 300, Choice C.

5. B: We are looking for the section where we would find books on Judaism, which is a religion. Choice A is about philosophy and psychology; this is not relevant, nor is Choice C which covers social sciences. Choice D, history, could be helpful, but overall, Judaism is a religion. Thus, Choice B, religion, is the correct answer.

6. B: Samuel wants to write an academic paper based on his 24 students. His best students come from homes where parental supervision is minimal, while the worst come from parents with extensive involvement. His conclusion is counterintuitive and probably the result of a small sample size. Choices A and D having to do with bias, is not the issue, nor is Choice C. Samuel's experience with these students is not applicable to students in general; rather, it is a tiny sample size relative to the millions of school children in the United States. The correct answer is B since the sample contains too few members to make meaningful claims applicable to a large group.

7. B: The passage indicates that Annabelle has a fear of going outside into the daylight. Thus *heliophobia* must refer to a fear of bright lights or sunlight. Choice B is the only answer that describes this.

8. C: After removing the first and last letter, *OATHIN* remains. Next, we eliminate all the vowels, except *I*, to get *THIN*. Finally, we remove the *H* to get *TIN*; thus, Choice C is the correct answer.

9. C: The answer we seek has both the most detailed and objective information. Choice *A* describing a television commercial with a dramatized reenactment is not particularly detailed. Choice *B*, a notice to the public informing them of additional drinking and driving units on patrol, is not detailed and objective information. Choice *D*, a highway bulletin, does not present the type of information required. Choice *C* is the correct answer. The number of incidents and their relationship to a possible cause are both detailed and objective information.

10. C: We are looking for an inference—a conclusion that is reached on the basis of evidence and reasoning—from the passage that will likely explain why the famous children's author did not achieve her usual success with the new genre (despite the book's acclaim). Choice *A* is wrong because the statement is false according to the passage. Choice *B* is wrong because, although the passage says the author has a graduate degree on the subject, it would be an unrealistic leap to infer that she is the foremost expert on Antebellum America. Choice *D* is wrong because there is nothing in the passage to lead us to infer that people generally prefer a children's series to historical fiction. In contrast, Choice *C* can be logically inferred since the passage speaks of the great success of the children's series and the declaration that the fame of the author's name causes the children's books to "fly off the shelves." Thus, she did not receive any bump from her name since she published the historical novel under a pseudonym, and Choice *C* is correct.

11. B: Narrative, Choice *A*, means a written account of connected events. Think of narrative writing as a story. Choice *C*, expository writing, generally seeks to explain or describe some phenomena, whereas Choice *D*, technical writing, includes directions, instructions, and/or explanations. This passage is definitely persuasive writing, which hopes to change someone's beliefs based on an appeal to reason or emotion. The author is aiming to convince the reader that smoking is terrible. They use health, price, and beauty in their argument against smoking, so Choice *B*, persuasive, is the correct answer.

12. B: The author is clearly opposed to tobacco. He cites disease and deaths associated with smoking. He points to the monetary expense and aesthetic costs. Choice *A* is wrong because alternatives to smoking are not even addressed in the passage. Choice *C* is wrong because it does not summarize the passage but rather is just a premise. Choice *D* is wrong because, while these statistics are a premise in the argument, they do not represent a summary of the piece. Choice *B* is the correct answer because it states the three critiques offered against tobacco and expresses the author's conclusion.

13. C: We are looking for something the author would agree with, so it will almost certainly be anti-smoking or an argument in favor of quitting smoking. Choice *A* is wrong because the author does not speak against means of cessation. Choice *B* is wrong because the author does not reference other substances, but does speak of how addictive nicotine, a drug in tobacco, is. Choice *D* is wrong because the author certainly would not encourage reducing taxes to encourage a reduction of smoking costs, thereby helping smokers to continue the habit. Choice *C* is correct because the author is definitely attempting to persuade smokers to quit smoking.

14. D: Here, we are looking for an opinion of the author's rather than a fact or statistic. Choice *A* is wrong because quoting statistics from the Centers of Disease Control and Prevention is stating facts, not opinions. Choice *B* is wrong because it expresses the fact that cigarettes sometimes cost more than a few gallons of gas. It would be an opinion if the author said that cigarettes were not affordable. Choice *C* is incorrect because yellow stains are a known possible adverse effect of smoking. Choice *D* is correct as an opinion because smell is subjective. Some people might like the smell of smoke, they might not have working olfactory senses, and/or some people might not find the smell of smoke akin to "pervasive nastiness," so this is the expression of an opinion. Thus, Choice *D* is the correct answer.

15. D: Outspending other countries on education could have other benefits, but there is no reference to this in the passage, so Choice *A* is incorrect. Choice *B* is incorrect because the author does not mention corruption. Choice *C* is incorrect because there is nothing in the passage stating that the tests are not genuinely representative. Choice *D* is accurate because spending more money has not brought success. The United States already spends the most money, and the country is not excelling on these tests. Choice *D* is the correct answer.

16. A: The guide words indicate that all of the other words on the page will be found between those words when listed alphabetically. The two guide words are *kingcraft* and *klieg light*, so the correct answer will fit between the two when ordering them alphabetically. Choice *B*, *knead*, comes after *klieg light*; Choice *C*, *kinesthesia*, and Choice *D*, *kickback*, both come before *kingcraft*. The correct answer is Choice *A*, *kleptomania*.

17. C: A primary source is an artifact, document, recording, or other source of information that is created at the time under study. Think of a primary source as the original representation of the information. In contrast, secondary sources make conclusions or draw inferences based on primary sources, as well as other secondary sources. Choice *A*, therefore, a critic's summary and review of a new book is a secondary source; additionally, the book itself may be a secondary source. Choice *B*, a table of contents, is a secondary source since it refers to other information. Choice *D*, a news article quoting research, is also a secondary source. Therefore, a report of the groundbreaking research itself, Choice *C*, is correct.

18. D: Cynthia needs to select the meal with the least vegetarian options. Although the breakfast menu, Choice *A*, includes bacon, there is also coffee, tea, French toast, and eggs available. Choice *B*, lunch, includes an option for vegetarian sandwiches along with the French fries and baked beans. The cocktail hour, Choice *C*, does not contain meat or fish. In contrast, the dinner is a vegetarian's nightmare: nothing suitable is offered. Thus, dinner, Choice *D*, is the best answer.

19. D: Although Washington is from a wealthy background, the passage does not say that his wealth led to his republican ideals, so Choice *A* is not supported. Choice *B* also does not follow from the passage. Washington's warning against meddling in foreign affairs does not mean that he would oppose wars of every kind, so Choice *B* is wrong. Choice *C* is also unjustified since the author does not indicate that Alexander Hamilton's assistance was absolutely necessary. Choice *D* is correct because the farewell address clearly opposes political parties and partisanship. The author then notes that presidential elections often hit a fever pitch of partisanship. Thus, it is follows that George Washington would not approve of modern political parties and their involvement in presidential elections.

20. A: The author finishes the passage by applying Washington's farewell address to modern politics, so the purpose probably includes this application. Choice *B* is wrong because George Washington is already a well-established historical figure; furthermore, the passage does not seek to introduce him. Choice *C* is wrong because the author is not fighting a common perception that Washington was merely a military hero. Choice *D* is wrong because the author is not convincing readers. Persuasion does not correspond to the passage. Choice *A* states the primary purpose.

21. D: Choice *A* is wrong because the last paragraph is not appropriate for a history textbook. Choice *B* is false because the piece is not a notice or announcement of Washington's death. Choice *C* is clearly false because it is not fiction, but a historical writing. Choice *D* is correct. The passage is most likely to appear in a newspaper editorial because it cites information relevant and applicable to the present day, a popular format in editorials.

22. B: The scientist and politician largely disagree, but the question asks for a point where the two are in agreement. The politician would not concur that burning fossil fuels causes global temperatures to rise; thus, Choice *A* is wrong. He would not agree with Choice *C* suggesting that countries must revisit their energy policies. By inference from the given information, the scientist would likely not concur that earth's climate naturally goes through warming and cooling cycles; so Choice *D* is incorrect. However, both the scientist and politician would agree that global temperatures are increasing. The reason for this is in dispute. The politician thinks it is part of the earth's natural cycle; the scientist thinks it is from the burning of fossil fuels. However, both acknowledge an increase, so Choice *B* is the correct answer.

23. D: Raul wants a book that describes how and why ancient Egyptians built the Great Pyramid of Giza. Choice *A* is incorrect because it focuses more generally on Giza as a whole, rather than the Great Pyramid itself. Choice *B* is close but incorrect because it is an autobiography that will largely focus on the archaeologist's life. Choice *C* is wrong because it focuses on hieroglyphics; it is not directly on point. Choice *D*, the book directly covering the building of the Great Pyramids, should be most helpful.

24. D: The passage does not proceed in chronological order since it begins by pointing out Leif Erikson's explorations in America so Choice *A* does not work. Although the author compares and contrasts Erikson with Christopher Columbus, this is not the main way the information is presented; therefore, Choice *B* does not work. Neither does Choice *C* because there is no mention of or reference to cause and effect in the passage. However, the passage does offer a conclusion (Leif Erikson deserves more credit) and premises (first European to set foot in the New World and first to contact the natives) to substantiate Erikson's historical importance. Thus, Choice *D* is correct.

25. C: Choice *A* is wrong because it describes facts: Leif Erikson was the son of Erik the Red and historians debate Leif's date of birth. These are not opinions. Choice *B* is wrong; that Erikson called the land Vinland is a verifiable fact as is Choice *D* because he did contact the natives almost 500 years before Columbus. Choice *C* is the correct answer because it is the author's opinion that Erikson deserves more credit. That, in fact, is his conclusion in the piece, but another person could argue that Columbus or another explorer deserves more credit for opening up the New World to exploration. Rather than being an incontrovertible fact, it is a subjective value claim.

26. B: Choice *A* is wrong because the author aims to go beyond describing Erikson as a mere legendary Viking. Choice *C* is wrong because the author does not focus on Erikson's motivations, let alone name the spreading of Christianity as his primary objective. Choice *D* is wrong because it is a premise that Erikson contacted the natives 500 years before Columbus, which is simply a part of supporting the author's conclusion. Choice *B* is correct because, as stated in the previous answer, it accurately identifies the author's statement that Erikson deserves more credit than he has received for being the first European to explore the New World.

27. B: Choice *A* is wrong because the author is not in any way trying to entertain the reader. Choice *D* is wrong because he goes beyond a mere suggestion; "suggest" is too vague. Although the author is certainly trying to alert the readers (make them aware) of Leif Erikson's underappreciated and unheralded accomplishments, the nature of the writing does not indicate the author would be satisfied with the reader merely knowing of Erikson's exploration (Choice *C*). Rather, the author would want the reader to be informed about it, which is more substantial (Choice *B*).

28. D: Choice *A* is wrong because the author never addresses the Vikings' state of mind or emotions. Choice *B* is wrong because the author does not elaborate on Erikson's exile and whether he would have become an explorer if not for his banishment. Choice *C* is wrong because there is not enough information to support this premise. It is unclear whether Erikson informed the King of Norway of his finding. Although it is true that the King did not send a follow-up expedition, he could have simply chosen not to expend the resources after receiving Erikson's news. It is not possible to logically infer whether Erikson told him. Choice *D* is correct because there are two examples—Leif Erikson's date of birth and what happened during the encounter with the natives—of historians having trouble pinning down important dates in Viking history.

29. C: The question asks which of the battles in the chart that are listed in this question had more Confederate casualties than Union casualties. There were more Confederate casualties than Union casualties at the Battles of Gettysburg and Atlanta. Of the two, only Atlanta is listed as an answer choice. Thus, C, Atlanta, is the correct answer.

30. D: The question is asking you to find where the dates are located in the table and to identify the earliest battle. Answer D, Shiloh, occurred in April 1862 and no other battle listed on the table happened until May 1863.

31. A: Robert E. Lee led the Confederate army in all battles listed on the table, except Shiloh and Atlanta. Shiloh is not listed in the question, therefore Atlanta, option A, is the correct answer.

32. A: This question is asking you to compare the Union and Confederate casualties and find the one listed where the Union casualties most exceeded the Confederate ones. At Cold Harbor, there were approximately 8,142 more Union casualties than Confederate. At Chancellorsville, there were approximately 3,844 more Union casualties. At Atlanta the number of Confederate casualties exceeded the Union number, so it cannot be the correct answer. At Shiloh there were approximately 2,378 more Union casualties. Thus, the number of Union casualties most greatly exceeding the Confederate number was at Cold Harbor, making *A*, Cold Harbor, the correct answer.

33. D: To calculate the total American casualties, we combine the Union and Confederate casualties since it was a civil war with Americans on both sides. There were approximately 51,112 (Union + Confederate losses) American casualties at Gettysburg; thus, the correct answer will be a battle with approximately 25,556 casualties which is half of that number. Shiloh is the closest with a total of 23,716 casualties, making D the correct answer.

34. C: The correct answer choice is C, *1910*. There are two ways to arrive at the correct answer. You could find the four answer choices on the graph, or you could have identified that the population never dips at any point. Thus, the correct answer needs to be the only answer choice that is earlier in time than the others, Choice *C*.

35. D: The population increased the most between 1990 and 2010. The question is asking you to identify the rate of change for each interval. Between 1930 and 1950, the population increased by approximately 28 million. Between 1950 and 1970, the population increased by approximately 52 million. Between 1970 and 1990, the population increased by approximately 45 million. Between 1990 and 2010, the population increased by approximately 60 million. Thus, D is the correct answer. The slope is also the steepest in this interval, which represents its higher increase.

36. B: Choice *A* is irrelevant as Chapter 5 is for outdoor activities as a whole and not only for ones that start with a particular letter. Choice *C* brings up an omission, not a potential inconsistency; furthermore, Chapter 5 does not have to include all outdoor activities. Choice *D* points out a possible inconsistency; however, it would only be an inconsistency if all the other sections contained tips. The camping section does not contain any tips. Choice *B* is the correct answer because every segment except of cycling contains a section about equipment or gear.

37. B: Primary producers make up the base of the food chain, so the correct answer will be in the level just above: a primary consumer. The cobra, wild dog, and aardvark are all secondary consumers. The gazelle is a primary consumer, so B is the correct answer.

38. A: According to the passage preceding the food chain, the apex predators do not have natural predators. So, the question is really asking which of the answer choices is an apex predator. The cobra, mongoose, and aardvark are all secondary consumers. The vulture is an apex predator; thus, a vulture has no natural predators, making A the correct answer.

39. D: A mongoose is a secondary consumer; thus, the mongoose consumes primary consumers. The shrub is a primary producer. The aardvark is a secondary consumer. The vulture is an apex predator. The mouse is a primary consumer, so Choice *D* is the correct answer.

40. D: This question is testing whether you realize how a timeline illustrates information in chronological order from left to right. "Started school for the deaf" is fourth on the timeline from the left, which means that it is the fourth event on the timeline. Thus, Choice *D* is the correct answer.

41. B: This question is asking you to determine the length of time between the pairs of events listed as answer choices. Events in timelines are arranged proportional to time. To determine the answer to this question, one must find the largest space between two events. Visually, this can be seen between the events of befriending Helen Keller and dying in Canada. Thus, choice B is the correct answer.

42. C: This question is testing whether you can discern accurate conclusions from a timeline. Although the incorrect answer choices can seem correct, they cannot be confirmed from the information presented on the timeline. Choice *A* is incorrect; while it may be reasonable to assume that the timeline documents all major life events, we do not know for certain that Bell did not engage in any notable activities after founding the National Geographic Society. Choice *B* is incorrect because the timeline does not confirm that the school was in Canada; Bell actually started it in the United States. Choice *D* is incorrect because nothing on the timeline shows causation between the two events. According to the timeline, answer choice "C" is the only verifiable statement based on the timeline. Thus, choice C is the correct answer.

43. B: The founding of the school is the event listed farthest to the right of the events in the answer choices. This means it occurred most recently. Thus, D is the correct answer.

44. B: Choice *A*, Choice *C*, and Choice *D* all relate facts but do not present the kind of general statement that would serve as an effective summary or conclusion. Choice *B* is correct.

45. B: Choice *A* uses similar language, but it is not the main point of disagreement. The reporter calls the loss devastating, and there's no reason to believe that the coach would disagree with this assessment. Eliminate this choice.

Choice *B* is strong since both passages mention the at-bats with runners in scoring position. The reporter asserts that the team lost due to the team failing to get such a hit. In contrast, the coach identifies several other reasons for the loss, including fielding and pitching errors. Additionally, the coach disagrees that the team even needed a hit in those situations.

Choice C is mentioned by the coach, but not by the reporter. It is unclear whether the reporter would agree with this assessment. Eliminate this choice.

Choice D is mentioned by the coach but not by the reporter. It is not stated whether the reporter believes that the team deserved to win. Eliminate this choice.

Therefore, Choice B is the correct answer.

46. D: Choice D correctly summarizes Frost's theme of life's journey and the choices one makes. While Choice A can be seen as an interpretation, it is a literal one and is incorrect. Literal is not symbolic. Choice B presents the idea of good and evil as a theme, and the poem does not specify this struggle for the traveler. Choice C is a similarly incorrect answer. Love is not the theme.

47. D: Choice A is irrelevant. The argument does not address whether Kimmy deserves her fame. Eliminate this choice.

Choice B restates a premise. Kimmy starring in an extremely popular movie is only one piece of the argument. It is not the main purpose. Eliminate this choice.

Choice C also restates a premise, and it is incorrect for the same reasons as Choice B. Eliminate this choice.

Choice D accurately expresses the argument's conclusion, and it best describes the argument's primary purpose. The argument concludes that Kimmy is a world famous actress. Choice D is the best expression of the argument's purpose.

Therefore, Choice D is the correct answer.

48. D: Choice A is clearly incorrect. The argument does not start with a conclusion. Eliminate this choice.

Choice B is incorrect. Although the argument states a universal rule—the top salesman is always a company's best employee—it does not argue that Dwight is the exception. Eliminate this choice.

Choice C is fairly strong. The argument does state several facts and offers a conclusion based on those facts. Leave this choice for now.

Choice D looks extremely promising. The argument first states several facts—Dwight works at a mid-sized regional tech company and leads the company in sales—then states a rule. Lastly, the argument applies the facts to the rule and concludes that Dwight is the best employee. This is a better fit than Choice C since it includes the rule and its application.

Therefore, Choice D is the correct answer.

49. D: To enlighten the audience on the habits of sun-fish and their hatcheries. Choice A is incorrect because although the Adirondack region is mentioned in the text, there is no cause or effect relationships between the region and fish hatcheries depicted here. Choice B is incorrect because the text does not have an agenda, but rather is meant to inform the audience. Finally, Choice C is incorrect because the text says nothing of how sun-fish mate.

50. B: The word *wise* in this passage most closely means *manner*. Choices A and C are synonyms of *wise*; however, they are not relevant in the context of the text. Choice D, *ignorance*, is opposite of the word *wise*, and is therefore incorrect.

51. A: Fish at the stage of development where they are capable of feeding themselves. Even if the word *fry* isn't immediately known to the reader, the context gives a hint when it says "until the fry are hatched out and are sufficiently large to take charge of themselves."

52. C: The passage is told in chronological order, detailed the steps the family took to adopt their dog. The narrator mentions that Robin's physical exam and lab work confirmed she was healthy before discussing that they brought her to the vet to evaluate her health. It is illogical that lab work would confirm good health prior to an appointment with the vet, when presumably, the lab work would be collected.

53. D: The graph displaying the percentage of weekly homework assignments Marco completed clearly shows a recent decline. It is likely that test performance may suffer without adequate practice, which is one of the primary purposes of homework assignments. Choice *A*, the email, would not necessarily substantiate a poor mark because the absences have not yet occurred and therefore, would not factor into the prior exam. Choice *B*, the graph of test scores simply demonstrates that indeed his score was lower than it had been. Choice *C* is also incorrect because his absences have no obvious trend that would lend to decreased performance. They seem to have bounced around over the duration of the course.

Mathematics

1. A: Compare each numeral after the decimal point to figure out which overall number is greatest. In answers *A* (1.43785) and *C* (1.43592), both have the same tenths (4) and hundredths (3). However, the thousandths is greater in answer *A* (7), so *A* has the greatest value overall.

2. D: By grouping the four numbers in the answer into factors of the two numbers of the question (6 and 12), it can be determined that (3 x 2) x (4 x 3) = 6 x 12. Alternatively, each of the answer choices could be prime factored or multiplied out and compared to the original value. 6 × 12 has a value of 72 and a prime factorization of $2^3 \times 3^2$. The answer choices respectively have values of 64, 84, 108, and 72 and prime factorizations of 2^6, $2^2 \times 3 \times 7$, $2^2 \times 3^3$, and $2^3 \times 3^2$, so answer *D* is the correct choice.

3. C: The sum total percentage of a pie chart must equal 100%. Since the CD sales take up less than half of the chart and more than a quarter (25%), it can be determined to be 40% overall. This can also be measured with a protractor. The angle of a circle is 360°. Since 25% of 360 would be 90° and 50% would be 180°, the angle percentage of CD sales falls in between; therefore, it would be answer *C*.

4. B: Since $850 is the price *after* a 20% discount, $850 represents 80% of the original price. To determine the original price, set up a proportion with the ratio of the sale price (850) to original price (unknown) equal to the ratio of sale percentage:

$$\frac{850}{x} = \frac{80}{100}$$

(where *x* represents the unknown original price)

To solve a proportion, cross multiply the numerators and denominators and set the products equal to each other: (850)(100) = (80)(x). Multiplying each side results in the equation 85,000=80x.

To solve for x, divide both sides by 80: $\frac{85,000}{80} = \frac{80x}{80}$, resulting in $x=1062.5$. Remember that x represents the original price. Subtracting the sale price from the original price ($1062.50-$850) indicates that Frank saved $212.50.

5. A: To figure out which is largest, look at the first non-zero digits. Answer *B*'s first nonzero digit is in the hundredths place. The other three all have nonzero digits in the tenths place, so it must be *A*, *C*, or *D*. Of these, *A* has the largest first nonzero digit.

6. C: To solve for the value of b, both sides of the equation need to be equalized.

Start by cancelling out the lower value of -4 by adding 4 to both sides:

$$5b - 4 = 2b + 17$$

$$5b - 4 + 4 = 2b + 17 + 4$$

$$5b = 2b + 21$$

The variable *b* is the same on each side, so subtract the lower 2b from each side:

$$5b = 2b + 21$$

$$5b - 2b = 2b + 21 - 2b$$

$$3b = 21$$

Then divide both sides by 3 to get the value of *b*:

$$3b = 21$$

$$\frac{3b}{3} = \frac{21}{3}$$

$$b = 7$$

7. D: The total faculty is 15 + 20 = 35. So the ratio is 35:200. Then, divide both of these numbers by 5, since 5 is a common factor to both, with a result of 7:40.

8. C: The first step in solving this problem is expressing the result in fraction form. Separate this problem first by solving the division operation of the last two fractions. When dividing one fraction by another, invert or flip the second fraction and then multiply the numerator and denominator.

$$\frac{7}{10} \times \frac{2}{1} = \frac{14}{10}$$

Next, multiply the first fraction with this value:

$$\frac{3}{5} \times \frac{14}{10} = \frac{42}{50}$$

Decimals are expressions of 1 or 100%, so multiply both the numerator and denominator by 2 to get the fraction as an expression of 100.

$$\frac{42}{50} \times \frac{2}{2} = \frac{84}{100}$$

In decimal form, this would be expressed as 0.84.

9. C: 85% of a number means that number should be multiplied by 0.85: $0.85 \times 20 = \frac{85}{100} \times \frac{20}{1}$, which can be simplified to $\frac{17}{20} \times \frac{20}{1} = 17$. The answer is C.

10. D: This problem can be solved by setting up a proportion involving the given information and the unknown value. The proportion is:

$$\frac{21\ pages}{4\ nights} = \frac{140\ pages}{x\ nights}$$

Solving the proportion by cross-multiplying, the equation becomes $21x = 4 * 140$, where $x = 26.67$. Since it is not an exact number of nights, the answer is rounded up to 27 nights. Twenty-six nights would not give Sarah enough time.

11. B: Using the conversion rate, multiply the projected weight loss of 25 lb by $0.45\ \frac{kg}{lb}$ to get the amount in kilograms (11.25 kg).

12. D: First, subtract $1437 from $2334.50 to find Johnny's monthly savings; this equals $897.50. Then, multiply this amount by 3 to find out how much he will have (in three months) before he pays for his vacation: this equals $2692.50. Finally, subtract the cost of the vacation ($1750) from this amount to find how much Johnny will have left: $942.50.

13. B: Dividing by 98 can be approximated by dividing by 100, which would mean shifting the decimal point of the numerator to the left by 2. The result is 4.2 which rounds to 4.

14. B: To solve this correctly, keep in mind the order of operations with the mnemonic PEMDAS (Please Excuse My Dear Aunt Sally). This stands for Parentheses, Exponents, Multiplication, Division, Addition, Subtraction. Taking it step by step, solve the parentheses first:

$$4 \times 7 + (4)^2 \div 2$$

Then, apply the exponent:

$$4 \times 7 + 16 \div 2$$

Multiplication and division are both performed next:

$$28 + 8 = 36$$

15. C: The formula for the perimeter of a rectangle is P=2L+2W, where P is the perimeter, L is the length, and W is the width. The first step is to substitute all of the data into the formula:

$$36 = 2(12) + 2W$$

Simplify by multiplying 2x12:

$$36 = 24 + 2W$$

Simplifying this further by subtracting 24 on each side, which gives:

$$36-24 = 24-24+2W$$

$$12= 2W$$

Divide by 2:

$$6 = W$$

The width is 6 cm. Remember to test this answer by substituting this value into the original formula: 36 = 2(12) + 2(6).

16. D: To find the average of a set of values, add the values together and then divide by the total number of values. In this case, include the unknown value of what Dwayne needs to score on his next test, in order to solve it.

$$\frac{78 + 92 + 83 + 97 + x}{5} = 90$$

Add the unknown value to the new average total, which is 5. Then multiply each side by 5 to simplify the equation, resulting in:

$$78 + 92 + 83 + 97 + x = 450$$

$$350 + x = 450$$

$$x = 100$$

Dwayne would need to get a perfect score of 100 in order to get an average of at least 90.

Test this answer by substituting back into the original formula.

$$\frac{78 + 92 + 83 + 97 + 100}{5} = 90$$

17. D: For an even number of total values, the *median* is calculated by finding the *mean* or average of the two middle values once all values have been arranged in ascending order from least to greatest. In this case, $(92 + 83) \div 2$ would equal the median 87.5, answer *D*.

18. C: Follow the *order of operations* in order to solve this problem. Solve the parentheses first, and then follow the remainder as usual.

$$(6 \times 4) - 9$$

This equals $24 - 9$ or 15, answer *C*.

19. D: Three girls for every two boys can be expressed as a ratio: 3:2. This can be visualized as splitting the school into 5 groups: 3 girl groups and 2 boy groups. The number of students which are in each group can be found by dividing the total number of students by 5:

650 divided by 5 equals 1 part, or 130 students per group

To find the total number of girls, multiply the number of students per group (130) by how the number of girl groups in the school (3). This equals 390, answer *D*.

20. B: To solve this correctly, keep in mind the order of operations with the mnemonic PEMDAS (Please Excuse My Dear Aunt Sally). This stands for Parentheses, Exponents, Multiplication, Division, Addition, Subtraction. Taking it step by step, solve the parentheses first:

$$4 \times 7 + (4)^2 \div 2$$

Then, apply the exponent:

$$4 \times 7 + 16 \div 2$$

Multiplication and division are both performed next:

$$28 + 8 = 36$$

21. C: Kimberley worked 4.5 hours at the rate of \$10/h and 1 hour at the rate of \$12/h. The problem states that her pay is rounded to the nearest hour, so the 4.5 hours would round up to 5 hours at the rate of \$10/h. (5h)(\$10/h)+(1h)(\$12/h)= \$50+\$12= \$62.

22. D:

• $9x + x - 7 = 16 + 2x$	• Combine $9x$ and x.
• $10x - 7 = 16 + 2x$	•
• $10x - 7 + 7 = 16 + 2x + 7$	• Add 7 to both sides to remove (-7).
• $10x = 23 + 2x$	•
• $10x - 2x = 23 + 2x - 2x$	• Subtract 2x from both sides to move it to the other side of the equation.
• $8x = 23$	•
• $\dfrac{8x}{8} = \dfrac{23}{8}$	• Divide by 8 to get x by itself.
• $x = \dfrac{23}{8}$	•

23. C: The first step is to depict each number using decimals. $\dfrac{91}{100} = 0.91$

Multiplying both the numerator and denominator of $\dfrac{4}{5}$ by 20 makes it $\dfrac{80}{100}$ or 0.80; the closest approximation of $\dfrac{2}{3}$ would be $\dfrac{66}{100}$ or 0.66 recurring. Rearrange each expression in ascending order, as found in answer *C*.

24. B: First, calculate the difference between the larger value and the smaller value.

378 – 252 = 126

To calculate this difference as a percentage of the original value, and thus calculate the percentage *increase*, divide 126 by 252, then multiply by 100 to reach the percentage = 50%, answer *B*.

25. B: Add 3 to both sides to get $4x = 8$. Then divide both sides by 4 to get $x = 2$.

26. A: First simplify the larger fraction by separating it into two. When dividing one fraction by another, remember to *invert* the second fraction and multiply the two as follows:

$$\frac{5}{7} \times \frac{11}{9}$$

The resulting fraction $\frac{55}{63}$ cannot be simplified further, so this is the answer to the problem.

27. A: To calculate the range in a set of data, subtract the highest value with the lowest value. In this graph, the range of Mr. Lennon's students is 5, which can be seen physically in the graph as having the smallest difference compared with the other teachers between the highest value and the lowest value.

28. C: 300/80 =30/8 = 15/4 =3.75. But Bernard is only working full days, so he will need to work 4 days, since 3 days is not sufficient.

29. D: To calculate the circumference of a circle, use the formula $2\pi r$, where r equals the radius or half of the diameter of the circle and $\pi = 3.14 \dots$. Substitute the given information, $2\pi 5 = 31.4 \dots$, answer *D*.

30. A: Mean. An outlier is a data value that's either far above or below the majority of values in a sample set. The mean is the average of all values in the set. In a small sample, a very high or low number could greatly change the average. The median is the middle value when arranged from lowest to highest. Outliers would have no more of an effect on the median than any other value. Mode is the value that repeats most often in a set. Assuming that the same outlier doesn't repeat, outliers would have no effect on the mode of a sample set.

31. A: This vector indicates a positive relationship. A negative relationship would show points traveling from the top-left of the graph to the bottom-right. Exponential and logarithmic functions aren't linear (don't create a straight line), so these options could have been immediately eliminated.

32. A: The conversion can be obtained by setting up and solving the following equation:

$$4382 \, ft \, \times \frac{.3048 \, m}{1 \, ft} \times \frac{1 \, km}{1000 \, m} = 1.336 \, km$$

33. C: There is no verifiable relationship between the two variables. While it may seem to have somewhat of a positive correlation because of the last two data points: (5.6,8) and (6,7), you must also take into account the two data points before those (5,1) and (5.2, 2) that have low Y values despite high X values. Data with a normal distribution (Choice *A*) has an arc to it. This data does not.

34. D: The slope is given by the change in *y* divided by the change in *x*. Specifically, it's:

$$slope = \frac{y_2 - y_1}{x_2 - x_1}$$

The first point is (-5,-3) and the second point is (0,-1). Work from left to right when identifying coordinates. Thus the point on the left is point 1 (-5,-3) and the point on the right is point 2 (0,-1).

Now we need to just plug those numbers into the equation:

$$slope = \frac{-1 - (-3)}{0 - (-5)}$$

It can be simplified to:

$$slope = \frac{-1 + 3}{0 + 5}$$

$$slope = \frac{2}{5}$$

35. B: The figure is composed of three sides of a square and a semicircle. The sides of the square are simply added: 9 + 9 + 9 = 27 feet. The circumference of a circle is found by the equation C = 2πr. The radius is 4, so the circumference of the circle is 25.13 ft. Only half of the circle makes up the outer border of the figure (part of the perimeter) so half of 25.13 feet is 12.565 ft. Therefore, the total perimeter is: 27 ft + 12.565 ft = 39.565 ft. The other answer choices use the incorrect formula or fail to include all of the necessary sides.

36. A: The first step is to determine the unknown, which is in terms of the length, *l*.

The second step is to translate the problem into the equation using the perimeter of a rectangle, $P = 2l + 2w$. The width is the length minus 2 centimeters. The resulting equation is $2l + 2(l - 2) = 44$. The equation can be solved as follows:

• $2l + 2l - 4 = 44$	• Apply the distributive property on the left side of the equation
• $4l - 4 = 44$	• Combine like terms on the left side of the equation
• $4l = 48$	• Add 4 to both sides of the equation
• $l = 12$	• Divide both sides of the equation by 4

The length of the rectangle is 12 centimeters. The width is the length minus 2 centimeters, which is 10 centimeters. Checking the answers for length and width forms the following equation:

$$44 = 2(12) + 2(10)$$

The equation can be solved using the order of operations to form a true statement: $44 = 44$.

Science

1. A: When activated, B cells create antibodies against specific antigens. White blood cells are generated in yellow bone marrow, not cartilage. Platelets are not a type of white blood cell and are typically cell fragments produced by megakaryocytes. White blood cells are active throughout nearly all of one's life and have not been shown to specially activate or deactivate because of life events like puberty or menopause.

2. D: Mechanical digestion is physical digestion of food and tearing it into smaller pieces using force. This occurs in the stomach and mouth. Chemical digestion involves chemically changing the food and breaking it down into small organic compounds that can be utilized by the cell to build molecules. The salivary glands in the mouth secrete amylase that breaks down starch, which begins chemical digestion. The stomach contains enzymes such as pepsinogen/pepsin and gastric lipase, which chemically digest protein and fats, respectively. The small intestine continues to digest protein using the enzymes trypsin and chymotrypsin. It also digests fats with the help of bile from the liver and lipase from the pancreas. These organs act as exocrine glands because they secrete substances through a duct. Carbohydrates are digested in the small intestine with the help of pancreatic amylase, gut bacterial flora and fauna, and brush border enzymes like lactose. Brush border enzymes are contained in the towel-like microvilli in the small intestine that soak up nutrients.

3. D: The urinary system has many functions, the primary of which is removing waste products and balancing water and electrolyte concentrations in the blood. It also plays a key role in regulating ion concentrations, such as sodium, potassium, chloride, and calcium, in the filtrate. The urinary system helps maintain blood pH by reabsorbing or secreting hydrogen ions and bicarbonate as necessary. Certain kidney cells can detect reductions in blood volume and pressure and then can secrete renin to activate a hormone that causes increased reabsorption of sodium ions and water. This serves to raise blood volume and pressure. Kidney cells secrete erythropoietin under hypoxic conditions to stimulate red blood cell production. They also synthesize calcitriol, a hormone derivative of vitamin D3, which aids in calcium ion absorption by the intestinal epithelium.

4. B: The structure exclusively found in eukaryotic cells is the nucleus. Animal, plant, fungi, and protist cells are all eukaryotic. DNA is contained within the nucleus of eukaryotic cells, and they also have membrane-bound organelles that perform complex intracellular metabolic activities. Prokaryotic cells (archae and bacteria) do not have a nucleus or other membrane-bound organelles and are less complex than eukaryotic cells.

5. B: The cell structure responsible for cellular storage, digestion and waste removal is the lysosome. Lysosomes are like recycle bins. They are filled with digestive enzymes that facilitate catabolic reactions to regenerate monomers. The Golgi apparatus is designed to tag, package, and ship out proteins destined for other cells or locations. The centrioles typically play a large role only in cell division when they ratchet the chromosomes from the mitotic plate to the poles of the cell. The mitochondria are involved in energy production and are the powerhouses of the cell.

6. D: Density is found by dividing mass by volume:

$$density = \frac{mass}{volume}$$

The unit for mass (in this case grams) and the units for volume (in this case cm³) need to be combined together. They're combined as grams over volume since that's how they were set up in the equation:

$$d = \frac{14.3\ g}{5.4\ cm^3} = 2.65\ g/cm^3$$

7. D: Veins have valves, but arteries do not. Valves in veins are designed to prevent backflow, since they are the furthest blood vessels from the pumping action of the heart and steadily increase in volume (which decreases the available pressure). Capillaries diffuse nutrients properly because of their thin walls and high surface area and are not particularly dependent on positive pressure.

8. C: The blood leaves the right ventricle through a semi-lunar valve and goes through the pulmonary artery to the lungs. Any increase in pressure in the artery will eventually affect the contractibility of the right ventricle. Blood enters the right atrium from the superior and inferior venae cava veins, and blood leaves the right atrium through the tricuspid valve to the right ventricle. Blood enters the left atrium from the pulmonary veins carrying oxygenated blood from the lungs. Blood flows from the left atrium to the left ventricle through the mitral valve and leaves the left ventricle through a semi-lunar valve to enter the aorta.

9. D: Sodium bicarbonate, a very effective base, has the chief function to increase the pH of the chyme. Chyme leaving the stomach has a very low pH, due to the high amounts of acid that are used to digest and break down food. If this is not neutralized, the walls of the small intestine will be damaged and may form ulcers. Sodium bicarb is produced by the pancreas and released in response to pyloric stimulation so that it can neutralize the acid. It has little to no digestive effect.

10. D: A reflex arc is a simple nerve pathway involving a stimulus, a synapse, and a response that is controlled by the spinal cord—not the brain. The knee-jerk reflex is an example of a reflex arc. The stimulus is the hammer touching the tendon, reaching the synapse in the spinal cord by an afferent pathway. The response is the resulting muscle contraction reaching the muscle by an efferent pathway. None of the remaining processes is a simple reflex. Memories are processed and stored in the hippocampus in the limbic system. The visual center is located in the occipital lobe, while auditory processing occurs in the temporal lobe. The sympathetic and parasympathetic divisions of the autonomic nervous system control heart and blood pressure.

11. C: The lagging strand of DNA falls behind the leading strand because of its discontinuous synthesis. DNA helicase unzips the DNA helices so that synthesis can take place, and RNA primers are created by the RNA primase for the polymerases to attach to and build from. The lagging strand is synthesizing DNA in a direction that is hard for the polymerase to build, so multiple primers are laid down so that the entire length of DNA can be synthesized simultaneously, piecemeal. These short pieces of DNA being synthesized are known as Okazaki fragments and are joined together by DNA ligase.

12. A: The sternum is medial to the deltoid because it is much closer (typically right on) the midline of the body, while the deltoid is lateral at the shoulder cap. Superficial means that a structure is closer to the body surface and posterior means that it falls behind something else. For example, skin is superficial to bone and the kidneys are posterior to the rectus abdominus.

13. B: Ligaments connect bone to bone. Tendons connect muscle to bone. Both are made of dense, fibrous connective tissue (primary Type 1 collagen) to give strength. However, tendons are more organized, especially in the long axis direction like muscle fibers themselves, and they have more collagen. This arrangement makes more sense because muscles have specific orientations of their fibers, so they contract in somewhat predictable directions. Ligaments are less organized and more of a woven pattern because bone connections are not as organized as bundles or muscle fibers, so ligaments must have strength in multiple directions to protect against injury.

14. A: The three primary body planes are coronal, sagittal, and transverse. The coronal or frontal plane, named for the plane in which a corona or halo might appear in old paintings, divides the body vertically into front and back sections. The sagittal plane, named for the path an arrow might take when shot at the body, divides the body vertically into right and left sections. The transverse plane divides the body horizontally into upper or superior and lower or inferior sections. There is no medial plane, per se. The anatomical direction medial simply references a location close or closer to the center of the body than another location.

15. C: Although the lungs may provide some cushioning for the heart when the body is violently struck, this is not a major function of the respiratory system. Its most notable function is that of gas exchange for oxygen and carbon dioxide, but it also plays a vital role in the regulation of blood pH. The aqueous form of carbon dioxide, carbonic acid, is a major pH buffer of the blood, and the respiratory system directly controls how much carbon dioxide stays and is released from the blood through respiration. The respiratory system also enables vocalization and forms the basis for the mode of speech and language used by most humans.

16. A: The forebrain contains the cerebrum, the thalamus, the hypothalamus, and the limbic system. The limbic system is chiefly responsible for the perception of emotions through the amygdale, while the cerebrum interprets sensory input and generates movement. Specifically, the occipital lobe receives visual input, and the primary motor cortex in the frontal lobe is the controller of voluntary movement. The hindbrain, specifically the medulla oblongata and brain stem, control and regulate blood pressure and heart rate.

17. D: Germline mutations in eggs and sperm are permanent, can be on the chromosomal level, and will be inherited by offspring. Somatic mutations cannot affect eggs and sperm, and therefore are not inherited by offspring. Mutations of either kind are rarely beneficial to the individual, but do not necessarily harm them. Germline cells divide much more rapidly than do somatic cells, and a mutation in a sex cell would promulgate and affect many thousands of its daughter cells.

18. A: It is most likely asthma. Any of the answer choices listed can cause heavy breathing. A blood clot in the lung (*B*) could cause this, but this would be very uncommon for a child. Choices *C* and *D* can both be ruled out because the question mentions that it occurs even when the patient is relaxing. Hyperventilation is usually caused by a panic attack or some sort of physical activity. Asthma often develops during childhood. It would stand to reason then that the child may have not yet been diagnosed. While asthma attacks can be caused by exercise they can also occur when a person is not exerting themselves.

19. C: 2:9:10:4. These are the coefficients that follow the law of conservation of matter. The coefficient times the subscript of each element should be the same on both sides of the equation.

20. C: A catalyst functions to increase reaction rates by decreasing the activation energy required for a reaction to take place. Inhibitors would increase the activation energy or otherwise stop the reactants from reacting. Although increasing the temperature usually increases a reaction's rate, this is not true in all cases, and most catalysts do not function in this manner.

21. B: Biological catalysts are termed *enzymes*, which are proteins with conformations that specifically manipulate reactants into positions which decrease the reaction's activation energy. Lipids do not usually affect reactions, and cofactors, while they can aid or be necessary to the proper functioning of enzymes, do not make up the majority of biological catalysts.

22. B: Substances with higher amounts of hydrogen ions will have lower pHs, while substances with higher amounts of hydroxide ions will have higher pHs. Choice *A* is incorrect because it is possible to have an extremely strong acid with a pH less than 1, as long as its molarity of hydrogen ions is greater than 1. Choice *C* is false because a weak base is determined by having a pH lower than some value, not higher. Substances with pHs greater than 2 include anything from neutral water to extremely caustic lye. Choice *D* is false because a solution with a pH of 2 has ten times fewer hydrogen ions than a solution of pH 1.

23. A: Salts are formed from compounds that use ionic bonds. Disulfide bridges are special bonds in protein synthesis which hold the protein in their secondary and tertiary structures. Covalent bonds are strong bonds formed through the sharing of electrons between atoms and are typically found in organic molecules like carbohydrates and lipids. London dispersion forces are fleeting, momentary bonds which occur between atoms that have instantaneous dipoles but quickly disintegrate.

24. C: As in the last question, covalent bonds are special because they share electrons between multiple atoms. Most covalent bonds are formed between the elements H, F, N, O, S, and C, while hydrogen bonds are formed nearly exclusively between H and either O, N, or F. Covalent bonds may inadvertently form dipoles, but this does not necessarily happen. With similarly electronegative atoms like carbon and hydrogen, dipoles do not form, for instance. Crystal solids are typically formed by substances with ionic bonds like the salts sodium iodide and potassium chloride.

25. A: Gases like air will move and expand to fill their container, so they are considered to have an indefinite shape and indefinite volume. Liquids like water will move and flow freely, so their shapes change constantly, but do not change volume or density on their own. Solids change neither shape nor volume without external forces acting on them, so they have definite shapes and volumes.

26. A: The upper back has the one of the high densities of sweat glands of any area on the body. While palms, arms, and feet are often thought of as sweaty areas, they have relatively low amounts of sweat glands compared to other parts of the body. Remember that one of the purposes of sweat is thermoregulation, or controlling the temperature of the body. Regulating the temperature of one's core is more important than adjusting the temperature of one's extremities.

27. C: Nephrons are responsible for filtering blood. When functioning properly they allow blood cells and nutrients to go back into the bloodstream while sending waste to the bladder. However, nephrons can fail at doing this, particularly when blood flood to the kidneys is limited. The medulla (also called the renal medulla) (*A*) and the renal cortex (*D*) are both parts of the kidney but are not specifically responsible for filtering blood. The medulla is in the inner part of the kidney and contains the nephrons. The renal cortex is the outer part of the kidney. The heart (*B*) is responsible for pumping blood throughout the body rather than filtering it.

28. B: Ossification is the process by which cartilage, a soft, flexible substance is replaced by bone throughout the body. All humans regardless of age have cartilage, but cartilage in some areas goes away to make way for bones.

29. D: The outermost layer of the skin, the epidermis, consists of epithelial cells. This layer of skin is dead, as it has no blood vessels. Osteoclasts are cells that make up bones. Notice the prefix *Osteo-* which means bone. Connective tissue macrophage cells can be found in a variety of places, and dendritic cells are part of the lymphatic system.

30. C: mRNA is directly transcribed from DNA before being taken to the cytoplasm and translated by rRNA into a protein. tRNA transfers amino acids from the cytoplasm to the rRNA for use in building these proteins. siRNA is a special type of RNA which interferes with other strands of mRNA typically by causing them to get degraded by the cell rather than translated into protein.

31. B: Since the genotype is a depiction of the specific alleles that an organism's genes code for, it includes recessive genes that may or may not be otherwise expressed. The genotype does not have to name the proteins that its alleles code for; indeed, some of them may be unknown. The phenotype is the physical, visual manifestations of a gene, not the genotype. The genotype does not necessarily include any information about the organism's physical characters. Although some information about an organism's parents can be obtained from its genotype, its genotype does not actually show the parents' phenotypes.

32. C: One in four offspring (or 25%) will be short, so all four offspring cannot be tall. Although both of the parents are tall, they are hybrid or heterozygous tall, not homozygous. The mother's phenotype is for tall, not short. A Punnett square cannot determine if a short allele will die out. Although it may seem intuitive that the short allele will be expressed by lower numbers of the population than the tall allele, it still appears in 75% of the offspring (although its effects are masked in 2/3 of those). Besides, conditions could favor the recessive allele and kill off the tall offspring.

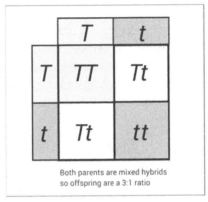

Both parents are mixed hybrids
so offspring are a 3:1 ratio

33. D: Evaporation takes place at the surface of a fluid while boiling takes place throughout the fluid. The liquid will boil when it reaches its boiling or vaporization temperature, but evaporation can happen due to a liquid's volatility. Volatile substances often coexist as a liquid and as a gas, depending on the pressure forced on them. The phase change from gas to liquid is condensation, and both evaporation and boiling take place in nature.

34. A: Human genes are strictly DNA and do not include proteins or amino acids. A human's genome and collection of genes will include even their recessive traits, mutations, and unused DNA.

35. C: Water's polarity lends it to be extremely cohesive and adhesive; this cohesion keeps its atoms very close together. Because of this, it takes a large amount of energy to melt and boil its solid and liquid forms. Phospholipid bilayers are made of nonpolar lipids and water, a polar liquid, cannot flow through it. Cell membranes use proteins called aquaporins to solve this issue and let water flow in and out. Fish breathe by capturing dissolved oxygen through their gills. Water can self-ionize, wherein it decomposes into a hydrogen ion (H^+) and a hydroxide ion (OH^-), but it cannot self-hydrolyze.

36. D: An isotope of an element has an atomic number equal to its number of protons, but a different mass number because of the additional neutrons. Even though there are differences in the nucleus, the behavior and properties of isotopes of a given element are identical. Atoms with different atomic numbers also have different numbers of protons and are different elements, so they cannot be isotopes.

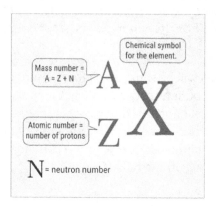

37. A: The neutrons and protons make up the nucleus of the atom. The nucleus is positively charged due to the presence of the protons. The negatively charged electrons are attracted to the positively charged nucleus by the electrostatic or Coulomb force; however, the electrons are not contained in the nucleus. The positively charged protons create the positive charge in the nucleus, and the neutrons are electrically neutral, so they have no effect. Radioactivity does not directly have a bearing on the charge of the nucleus.

38. C: To gather accurate data, the student must be able compare a participant's test score from round 1 with their test score from round 2. The differing levels of intellect among the participants means that comparing participants' test scores to those of other participants would be inaccurate. This requirement excludes choices A and D, which involve only one round of testing. The experiment must also involve different levels of sugar consumption from round 1 to round 2. In this way, the effects of different levels of sugar consumption can be seen on the same subjects. Thus, B is incorrect because the experiment provides for no variation of sugar consumption. C is the correct answer because it allows the student to compare each participant's test score from round 1 with their test score from round 2 after different level of sugar consumption.

39. D: The seminiferous tubules are responsible for sperm production. Had *testicles* been an answer choice, it would also have been correct since it houses the seminiferous tubules. The prostate gland (*A*) secretes enzymes that help nourish sperm after creation. The seminal vesicles (*B*) secrete some of the components of semen. The scrotum (*C*) is the pouch holding the testicles.

40. D: Based on this table, it can be reasoned that there is not a correlation between maintaining a calendar and GPA, since Student B never maintains a calendar but has the highest GPA of the cohort. Furthermore, it can be reasoned that there is a positive correlation between taking notes and GPA since the more notes a student takes, the higher the GPA they have Thus, Choice *D* is the correct answer. Choice *A* offers an absolute that cannot be proven based on this study; thus, it is incorrect. Choices B and C are incorrect because they have at least one incorrect correlation.

41. D: *D* is the correct answer because excess sunlight is a common cause of plant wilting. *A*, *B*, and *C* are all possible but unlikely to be a cause for wilting. Given that the test question asks for a *reasonable* explanation, *sunlight* is by far the most reasonable answer.

42. C: The parasympathetic nervous system is related to calm, peaceful times without stress that require no immediate decisions. It relaxes the fight-or-flight response, slows heart rate to a comfortable pace, and decreases bronchiole dilation to a normal size. The sympathetic nervous system, on the other hand, is in charge of the fight-or-flight response and works to increase blood pressure and oxygen absorption.

43. C: Neon, one of the noble gases, is chemically inert or not reactive because it contains eight valence electrons in the outermost shell. The atomic number is 10, with a 2.8 electron arrangement meaning that there are 2 electrons in the inner shell and the remaining 8 electrons in the outer shell. This is extremely stable for the atom, so it will not want to add or subtract any of its electrons and will not react under typical circumstances.

44. C: Because of the vast amounts of data that needed to be processed and analyzed, technological breakthroughs like innovations to the microprocessor were directly responsible for the ease of computing handled by the Human Genome Project. Although the sonogram and MRI technology are helpful to the healthcare industry in general, they would not have provided a great deal of help for sequencing and comprehending DNA data, in general. X-ray diffraction is a technique that helps visualize the structures of crystallized proteins, but cannot determine DNA bases with enough precision to help sequence DNA.

45. A: Many foods from developed countries are grown from plants which have been processed or bioengineered to include increased amounts of nutrients like vitamins and minerals that otherwise would be lost during manufacturing or are uncommon to the human diet. White rice, for example, is typically enriched with niacin, iron, and folic acid, while salt has been fortified with iodine for nearly a century. These help to prevent nutrition deficiencies. While it can be useful for fisheries to maintain models of fish populations so that they don't overfish their stock, this is not as immediately important to nutrition as are fortified and enriched foods. Although innovations to microscopes could lead to improved healthcare, this also has no direct effect on nutrition deficiency. Refrigerated train carts were historically a crucial invention around Civil War times and were used to transport meat and dairy products long distances without spoiling, but dietary deficiencies could be more easily remedied by supplying people with fortified foods containing those nutrients rather than spoilable meats.

46. C: The parathryroid gland impacts calcium levels by secreting parathyroid hormone (PTH). Osteotoid gland is not a real gland. The pineal gland regulates sleep by secreting melatonin, and the thymus gland focuses on immunity. *Thyroid* would also be a correct answer choice as it influences the levels of circulating calcium.

47. B: The most likely hypothesis that Anya is testing has something to with the pathophysiology of the bees, as she performed dissections on some of her samples. These dissections would be unnecessary if the bees were being killed off by another species, as the destruction of the hives would be obvious. As the deaths did not seem linked in any particular way geographically, it is also safe to assume that there was no correlation to cell phone towers, as maps of cell phone coverage would be readily available to her. If the pesticides were so toxic that the bees died on contact, then they wouldn't make it back to the hive to be available for her dissections or to drop off chemicals in the honey. The most likely of the choices is that parasites are killing off the bees, which would be easily communicable.

48. D: The law states that matter cannot be created or destroyed in a closed system. In this equation, there are the same number of molecules of each element on either side of the equation. Matter is not gained or lost, although a new compound is formed. As there are no ions on either side of the equation, no electrons are lost. The law prevents the hydrogen from losing mass and prevents oxygen atoms from being spontaneously spawned.

49. B: For measuring blood, we're looking for a unit that measures volume. Choices *A, B,* and *C,* are all measures of volume, but pounds (*D*) is a measure of weight. The correct answer is liters, as the average adult has about 5 liters of blood in their body. Blood can certainly be measured in ounces or milliliters; however, 5 liters is equal to 5,000 milliliters or 176 ounces. Thus, liters seems to be the more rational measuring unit.

50. B: The endocrine system's organs are glands which are spread throughout the body. The endocrine system itself does not connect the organs or transport the hormones they secrete. Rather, the various glands secrete the hormone into the bloodstream and lets the cardiovascular system pump it throughout the body. The other three body systems each include a network throughout the body:

- Cardiovascular system: veins and arteries
- Immune system: lymphatic vessels (it does also use the circulatory system)
- Nervous system: nerve networks

51. D: In the secondary immune response, suppressor T lymphocytes are activated to negate the potential risk of damage to healthy cells, brought on by an unchecked, overactive immune response. Choice *A* is incorrect because the activity is characteristic of the primary response, not the secondary response Choice *B* is incorrect because humeral immunity is mediated by antibodies produced by B, not T, lymphocytes. Choice *C* is wrong because the secondary response is faster than the primary response because the primary response entails the time-consuming process of macrophage activation.

52. C: Eosinophils, like neutrophils, basophils, and mast cells, are a type of leukocyte in a class called granulocytes. They are found underneath mucous membranes in the body and they primarily secrete destructive enzymes and defend against multicellular parasites like worms. Choice *A* describes basophils and mast cells, and Choice *B* and *D* describe neutrophils. Unlike neutrophils which are aggressive phagocytic cells, eosinophils have low phagocytic activity.

53. A: Keratin is a structural protein and it is the primary constituent of things like hair and nails. Choice *B* is incorrect antigens are immune proteins that help fight disease. Hormonal proteins are responsible for initiating the signal transduction cascade to regulate gene expression. Choice *C* is incorrect because channel proteins are transport proteins that help move molecules into and out of a cell. Marker proteins help identify or distinguish a cell. Lastly, Choice *D* is incorrect because actin, like myosin, is a motor protein because it is involved in the process of muscle contraction.

English and Language Usage

1. B: In choice B the word *Uncle* should not be capitalized, because it is not functioning as a proper noun. If the word named a specific uncle, such as *Uncle Jerry*, then it would be considered a proper noun and should be capitalized. Choice *A* correctly capitalizes the proper noun *East Coast*, and does not capitalize *winter*, which functions as a common noun in the sentence. Choice *C* correctly capitalizes the name of a specific college course, which is considered a proper noun. Choice *D* correctly capitalizes the proper noun *Jersey Shore*.

2. C: In choice C, *avid* is functioning as an adjective that modifies the word photographer. *Avid* describes the photographer Julia Robinson's style. The words *time* and *photographer* are functioning as nouns, and the word *capture* is functioning as a verb in the sentence. Other words functioning as adjectives in the sentence include, *local*, *business*, and *spare*, as they all describe the nouns they precede.

3. A: Choice *A* is correctly punctuated because it uses a semicolon to join two independent clauses that are related in meaning. Each of these clauses could function as an independent sentence. Choice *B* is incorrect because the conjunction is not preceded by a comma. A comma and conjunction should be used together to join independent clauses. Choice *C* is incorrect because a comma should only be used to join independent sentences when it also includes a coordinating conjunction such as *and* or *so*. Choice *D* does not use punctuation to join the independent clauses, so it is considered a fused (same as a run-on) sentence.

4. C: Choice *C* is a compound sentence because it joins two independent clauses with a comma and the coordinating conjunction *and*. The sentences in Choices B and D include one independent clause and one dependent clause, so they are complex sentences, not compound sentences. The sentence in Choice *A* has both a compound subject, *Alex and Shane*, and a compound verb, *spent and took*, but the entire sentence itself is one independent clause.

5. A: Choice *A* uses incorrect subject-verb agreement because the indefinite pronoun *neither* is singular and must use the singular verb form *is*. The pronoun *both* is plural and uses the plural verb form of *are*. The pronoun *any* can be either singular or plural. In this example, it is used as a plural, so the plural verb form *are* is used. The pronoun *each* is singular and uses the singular verb form *is*.

6. B: Choice *B* is correct because the pronouns *he* and *I* are in the subjective case. *He* and *I* are the subjects of the verb *like* in the independent clause of the sentence. Choice A, C, and D are incorrect because they all contain at least one objective pronoun (*me* and *him*). Objective pronouns should not be used as the subject of the sentence, but rather, they should come as an object of a verb. To test for correct pronoun usage, try reading the pronouns as if they were the only pronoun in the sentence. For example, *he* and *me* may appear to be the correct answer choices, but try reading them as the only pronoun.

He like[s] to go fishing...

Me like to go fishing...

When looked at that way, *me* is an obviously incorrect choice.

7. A: It is necessary to put a comma between the date and the year. It is also required to put a comma between the day of the week and the month. Choice *B* is incorrect because it is missing the comma between the day and year. Choice *C* is incorrect because it adds an unnecessary comma between the month and date. Choice *D* is missing the necessary comma between day of the week and the month.

8. D: *Discipline* and *perseverance* are both spelled correctly in choice *d*. These are both considered commonly misspelled words. One or both words are spelled incorrectly in choices A, B, and C.

9. D: In Choice D, the word function is a noun. While the word *function* can also act as a verb, in this particular sentence it is acting as a noun as the object of the preposition *at*. Choices A and B are incorrect because the word *function* cannot be used as an adjective or adverb.

10. C: Cacti is the correct plural form of the word *cactus*. Choice *A* (*tomatos*) includes an incorrect spelling of the plural of *tomato*. Both choice B (*analysis*) and choice D (*criterion*) are incorrect because they are in singular form. The correct plural form for these choices would be *criteria* and analyses.

11. B: Quotation marks are used to indicate something someone said. The example sentences feature a direct quotation that requires the use of double quotation marks. Also, the end punctuation, in this case a question mark, should always be contained within the quotation marks. Choice *A* is incorrect because there is an unnecessary period after the quotation mark. Choice *C* is incorrect because it uses single quotation marks, which are used for a quote within a quote. Choice *D* is incorrect because it places the punctuation outside of the quotation marks.

12. D: The prefix *trans* means across, beyond, over. Choices A, B, and C are incorrect because they are the meanings of other prefixes. Choice *A* is a meaning of the prefix *de*. Choice *B* is the meaning of the prefix *omni*. Choice *C* is one of the meanings of the prefix *pro*. The example words are helpful in determining the meaning of *trans*. All of the example words—*transfer, transact, translation, transport*—indicate something being *across, beyond,* or *over* something else. For example, *translation* refers to text going across languages. If no example words were given, you could think of words starting with *trans* and then compare their meanings to try to determine a common definition.

13. D: In choice D, the word *part* functions as an adjective that modifies the word *Irish*. Choices A and C are incorrect because the word *part* functions as a noun in these sentences. Choice *B* is incorrect because the word *part* functions as a verb.

14. C: *All of Shannon's family and friends* is the complete subject because it includes who or what is doing the action in the sentence as well as the modifiers that go with it. Choice *A* is incorrect because it only includes the simple subject of the sentence. Choices B and D are incorrect because they only include part of the complete subject.

15. D: Choice D directly addresses the reader, so it is in second person point of view. This is an imperative sentence since it issues a command; imperative sentences have an *understood you* as the subject. Choice *A* uses first person pronouns *I* and *my*. Choices B and C are incorrect because they use third person point of view.

16. A: The word *prodigious* is defined as very impressive, amazing, or large. In this sentence, the meaning can be drawn from the words *they became nervous about climbing its distant peak*, as this would be an appropriate reaction upon seeing a very large peak that's far in the distance. Choices B, C, and D do not accurately define the word *prodigious*, so they are incorrect.

17. D: Choice D correctly places a hyphen after the prefix *ex* to join it to the word *husband*. Words that begin with the prefixes *great, trans, ex, all,* and *self*, require a hyphen. Choices A and C place hyphens in words where they are not needed. *Beagle mix* would only require a hyphen if coming before the word *Henry*, since it would be serving as a compound adjective in that instance. Choice *B* contains hyphens that are in the correct place but are formatted incorrectly since they include spaces between the hyphens and the surrounding words.

18. C: Choice C is correct because quotation marks should be used for the title of a short work such as a poem. Choices A, B, and D are incorrect because the titles of novels, films, and newspapers should be placed in italics, not quotation marks.

19. A: This question focuses on the correct usage of the commonly confused word pairs of *it's/its* and *then/than*. *It's* is a contraction for *it is* or *it has*. *Its* is a possessive pronoun. The word *than* shows comparison between two things. *Then* is an adverb that conveys time. Choice *C* correctly uses *it's* and *than*. *It's* is a contraction for *it has* in this sentence, and *than* shows comparison between *work* and *rest*. None of the other answers choices use both of the correct words.

20. C: The suffix -fy means to make, cause, or cause to have. Choices A, B, and D are incorrect because they show meanings of other suffixes. Choice A shows the meaning of the suffix -ous. Choice B shows the meaning of the suffix –ist, and choice D shows the meaning of the suffix -age.

21. B: Dissatisfied and accommodations are both spelled correctly in Choice B. These are both considered commonly misspelled words. One or both words are spelled incorrectly in choices A, C, and D.

22. B: Choice B is an imperative sentence because it issues a command. In addition, it ends with a period, and an imperative sentence must end in a period or exclamation mark. Choice A is a declarative sentence that states a fact and ends with a period. Choice C is an exclamatory sentence that shows strong emotion and ends with an exclamation point. Choice D is an interrogative sentence that asks a question and ends with a question mark.

23. A: After and then are transitional words that indicate time or position. Choice B is incorrect because the words at, with, and to are used as prepositions in this sentence, not transitions. Choice C is incorrect because the words had and took are used as verbs in this sentence. In Choice D, a and the are used as articles in the sentence.

24. C: Choice C is a compound sentence because it joins two independent clauses—The baby was sick and I decided to stay home from work—with a comma and the coordinating conjunction so. Choices A, B, and D, are all simple sentences, each containing one independent clause with a complete subject and predicate. Choices A and D each contain a compound subject, or more than one subject, but they are still simple sentences that only contain one independent clause. Choice B contains a compound verb (more than one verb), but it's still a simple sentence.

25. A: Choice A includes all of the words functioning as nouns in the sentence. Choice B is incorrect because it includes the words final and academic, which are functioning as adjectives in this sentence. The word he makes Choice C incorrect because it is a pronoun. This example also includes the word library, which can function as a noun, but is functioning as an adjective modifying the word databases in this sentence. Choice D is incorrect because it leaves out the proper noun Robert.

26. C: The simple subject of this sentence, the word lots, is plural. It agrees with the plural verb form were. Choice A is incorrect, because the simple subject there, referring to the two constellations, is considered plural. It does not agree with the singular verb form is. In Choice B, the singular subject four, does not agree with the plural verb form needs. In Choice D the plural subject everyone does not agree with the singular verb form have.

27. B: Excellent and walking are adjectives modifying the noun tours. Rich is an adjective modifying the noun history, and brotherly is an adjective modifying the noun love. Choice A is incorrect because all of these words are functioning as nouns in the sentence. Choice C is incorrect because all of these words are functioning as verbs in the sentence. Choice D is incorrect because all of these words are considered prepositions, not adjectives.

28. D: The object pronouns her and me act as the indirect objects of the sentence. If me is in a series of object pronouns, it should always come last in the series. Choice A is incorrect because it uses subject pronouns she and I. Choice B is incorrect because it uses the subject pronoun she. Choice C uses the correct object pronouns, but they are in the wrong order.

29. A: In this example, a colon is correctly used to introduce a series of items. Choice *B* places an unnecessary comma before the word *because*. A comma is not needed before the word *because* when it introduces a dependent clause at the end of a sentence and provides necessary information to understand the sentence. Choice *C* is incorrect because it uses a semi-colon instead of a comma to join a dependent clause and an independent clause. Choice *D* is incorrect because it uses a colon in place of a comma and coordinating conjunction to join two independent clauses.

30. B: Choice *B* correctly uses the contraction for *you are* as the subject of the sentence, and it correctly uses the possessive pronoun *your* to indicate ownership of the jacket. It also correctly uses the adverb *there*, indicating place. Choice *A* is incorrect because it reverses the possessive pronoun *your* and the contraction for *you are*. It also uses the possessive pronoun *their* instead of the adverb *there*. Choice *C* is incorrect because it reverses *your* and *you're* and uses the contraction for *they are* in place of the adverb *there*. Choice *D* incorrectly uses the possessive pronoun *their* instead of the adverb *there*.

31. A: Only two of these suffixes, *–ize* and *–en*, can be used to form verbs, so *B* and *D* are incorrect. Those choices create adjectives. The suffix *–ize* means "to convert or turn into." The suffix *–en* means "to become." Because this sentence is about converting ideas into money, money + *–ize* or *monetize* is the most appropriate word to complete the sentence, so *C* is incorrect.

32. A: Slang refers to non-standard expressions that are not used in elevated speech and writing. Slang tends to be specific to one group or time period and is commonly used within groups of young people during their conversations with each other. Jargon refers to the language used in a specialized field. The vernacular is the native language of a local area, and a dialect is one form of a language in a certain region. Thus, *B*, *C*, and *D* are incorrect.

33. D: Colloquial language is that which is used conversationally or informally, in contrast to professional or academic language. While *ain't* is common in conversational English, it is a non-standard expression in academic writing. For college-bound students, high school should introduce them to the expectations of a college classroom, so *B* is not the best answer. Teachers should also avoid placing moral or social value on certain patterns of speech. Rather than teaching students that their familiar speech patterns are bad, teachers should help students learn when and how to use appropriate forms of expression, so *C* is wrong. *Ain't* is in the dictionary, so *A* is incorrect, both in the reason for counseling and in the factual sense.

Dear ATI TEAS Test Taker,

We would like to start by thanking you for purchasing this study guide for your ATI TEAS exam. We hope that we exceeded your expectations.

Our goal in creating this study guide was to cover all of the topics that you will see on the test. We also strove to make our practice questions as similar as possible to what you will encounter on test day. With that being said, if you found something that you feel was not up to your standards, please send us an email and let us know.

We would also like to let you know about other books in our catalog that may interest you.

HESI

This can be found on Amazon: amazon.com/dp/`

CEN

amazon.com/dp/1628454768

We have study guides in a wide variety of fields. If the one you are looking for isn't listed above, then try searching for it on Amazon or send us an email.

Thanks Again and Happy Testing!
Product Development Team
info@studyguideteam.com

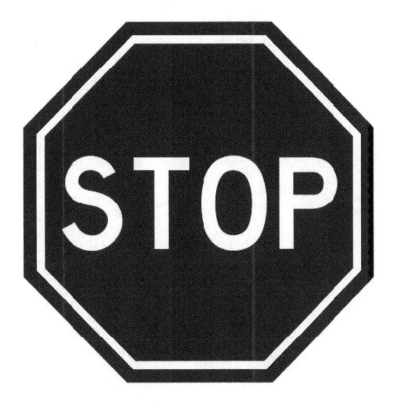

FREE Test Taking Tips DVD Offer

To help us better serve you, we have developed a Test Taking Tips DVD that we would like to give you for FREE. **This DVD covers world-class test taking tips that you can use to be even more successful when you are taking your test.**

All that we ask is that you email us your feedback about your study guide. Please let us know what you thought about it – whether that is good, bad or indifferent.

To get your **FREE Test Taking Tips DVD**, email freedvd@studyguideteam.com with "FREE DVD" in the subject line and the following information in the body of the email:

   a. The title of your study guide.

   b. Your product rating on a scale of 1-5, with 5 being the highest rating.

   c. Your feedback about the study guide. What did you think of it?

   d. Your full name and shipping address to send your free DVD.

If you have any questions or concerns, please don't hesitate to contact us at freedvd@studyguideteam.com.

Thanks again!

CPSIA information can be obtained
at www.ICGtesting.com
Printed in the USA
LVHW10s1802020918
588937LV00006BA/247/P